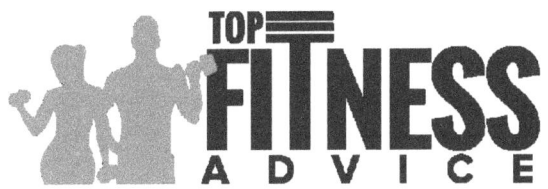

GYM BIBLE

The #1 Weight Training & Bodybuilding Guide for Men – Build Real Strength & Transform Your Body

Bruce Harlow

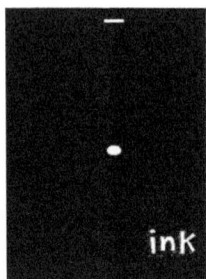

First published in 2017 by Venture Ink Publishing

Copyright © Top Fitness Advice 2019

All rights reserved.

No part of this book may be reproduced in any form without permission in writing from the author. No part of this publication may be reproduced or transmitted in any form or by any means, mechanic, electronic, photocopying, recording, by any storage or retrieval system, or transmitted by email without the permission in writing from the author and publisher.

Requests to the publisher for permission should be addressed to publishing@ventureink.co

For more information about the contents of this book or questions to the author, please contact Bruce Harlow at bruce@topfitnessadvice.com

Disclaimer

This book provides wellness management information in an informative and educational manner only, with information that is general in nature and that is not specific to you, the reader. The contents of this book are intended to assist you and other readers in your personal wellness efforts. Consult your physician regarding the applicability of any information provided in this book to you.

Nothing in this book should be construed as personal advice or diagnosis, and must not be used in this manner. The information provided about conditions is general in nature. This information does not cover all possible uses, actions, precautions, side-effects, or interactions of medicines, or medical procedures. The information in this book should not be considered as complete and does not cover all diseases, ailments, physical conditions, or their treatment.

You should consult with your physician before beginning any exercise, weight loss, or health care program. This book should not be used in place of a call or visit to a competent health-care professional. You should consult a health care professional before adopting any of the suggestions in this book or before drawing inferences from it.

Any decision regarding treatment and medication for your condition should be made with the advice and consultation of a qualified health care professional. If you have, or suspect you have, a health-care problem, then you should immediately contact a qualified health care professional for treatment.

No Warranties: The author and publisher don't guarantee or warrant the quality, accuracy, completeness, timeliness, appropriateness or suitability of the information in this book, or of any product or services referenced in this book.

The information in this book is provided on an "as is" basis and the author and publisher make no representations or warranties of any kind with respect to this information. This book may contain inaccuracies, typographical errors, or other errors.

Liability Disclaimer: The publisher, author, and other parties involved in the creation, production, provision of information, or delivery of this book specifically disclaim any responsibility, and shall not be held liable for any damages, claims, injuries, losses, liabilities, costs, or obligations including any direct, indirect, special, incidental, or consequences damages (collectively known as "Damages") whatsoever and howsoever caused, arising out of, or in connection with the use or misuse of the site and the information contained within it, whether such Damages arise in contract, tort, negligence, equity, statute law, or by way of other legal theory.

Table of Contents

Disclaimer — 3

Who Is This Book For? — 7

What Will This Book Teach You? — 9

Introduction — 11

Chapter 1: Basic Principles of Weight Training — 15

Chapter 2: Elements of an Effective Weight Training Program — 21

Chapter 3: Setting Your Goals — 25

Chapter 4: Safety First — 37

Chapter 5: Killer Weight Training Programs Part 1: Training for Appearance — 47

Chapter 6: Killer Weight Training Programs Part 2: Training for Performance — 61

Chapter 7: The Moves — 75

Chapter 8: Nutrition — 133

Conclusion — 141

Final Words — 143

Would you prefer to listen to my book, rather than read it?

Download the audiobook version for free!

If you go to the special link below and sign up to Audible as a new customer, you can get the audiobook version of my book completely free.

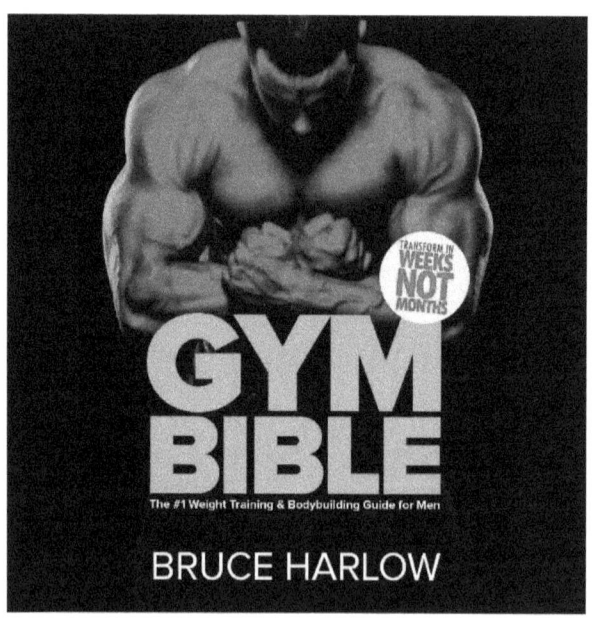

Go here to get your audiobook version for free:

TopFitnessAdvice.com/go/GymBible

Who Is This Book For?

This book is for the gym enthusiast looking for fitness hacks that will positively change the way he trains his body.

Do you have less than a month to prepare for an outing where you plan to flaunt your beach-ready body? Are you a returning athlete who just came from a long slump or just recovered from an injury and want to splash back into performance shape in no time?

Have you ever walked into the gym with absolutely no idea what you're going to do? Maybe you tried to imitate an exercise that you saw from another fella and you thought it was cool, but you didn't really know what it was for?

Perhaps you've always known what to do. You've researched it on the internet, you saw it on YouTube, you talked to your instructor, and you did exactly what you were told to do.

Yet weeks later, you still don't want to admit to your friends that you started lifting weights. Why? Because they wouldn't believe you - because the results aren't there yet!

And you're going to wait out until a couple of months before anyone would start to notice any change in your body, hopefully before you get frustrated waiting for the results.

Are you planning to partake in a lifelong commitment to fitness through weight training?

If you are the type of person who doesn't want to waste time and energy in fruitless endeavors, you love your body, you want to look good, or you answered yes to any of the questions above – this book is for you.

What Will This Book Teach You?

The *Gym Bible* contains the ultimate cheat codes to a successful weight training program! It is a comprehensive guide that tells you all you need to know about weight training and how to maximize your body's potential using this training discipline – minus the myths. Cut the time and see the results almost immediately.

Weight training is not just a discipline. It is also an exact science. You need to be fully equipped with the proper and sufficient knowledge of its science and how you can apply it to your own workouts in order to be successful. Follow this book, and expect to see results in weeks, not months.

The book contains a wide spectrum of information on weight training – from basic to advanced, but it is compressed into only the materials you need in order to become successful in its practice.

It contains exercises, nutritional guide, and sample training programs from beginner to advanced level, and a few tips on preventing and dealing with injuries – all written in easy to understand, non-academic format that you will enjoy reading till the very end. It's like having a friendly gym instructor coaching you through this book.

Some of the techniques and knowledge you will find in this book go against conventional "old school" wisdom of weight training – traditional knowledge that was proven to be ineffective. I only included modern, scientifically proven principles that make weight training the bread and butter of successful athletes and every fitness enthusiast.

Yes, the cheat codes are out! And it's right here.

Introduction

The practice of weight training without a thorough understanding of its principles is an exercise in futility. What separates fast developers from slow developers are not just genetics – it is also who does it right and who doesn't.

In weight training, if you know what you are doing, you can expect results. The better you know, the faster the results. The quality of your training also determines the quality of your development.

Of course, genetics play a big factor in our physical development and determines the extent of our full potential. But in order to achieve this full potential, there are controllable variables that we can tweak to maximize our nature-given physical talents and appearance.

Most individuals who do weight training are doing it either to improve their athletic abilities, improve how their body looks, or simply maintain their physical fitness. Whatever your goals are, there are tools that will help you get there, and knowledge is the primary of these tools.

These fitness hacks will help you achieve your goals in the shortest time possible. Get there, and get there fast.

Did You Know You Are MOST Likely Burning Fat Too SLOW?

Discover The Most POWERFUL Method to Start Burning Fat Up to 400% Faster!

For this month only, you can get Bruce's best-selling & most popular book absolutely free – *The Most Powerful Method to Burn Fat Up to 400% Faster!*

Get Your FREE Copy Here:
TopFitnessAdvice.com/Download

Discover exactly what you need to do to **put your metabolism into hyperdrive** and have your **fat melt away effortlessly**. And learn the biological "hacks" that have been scientifically proven to **boost the rate that your body burns fat by up to 400%.** With this book, readers were able to reach their fitness goals significantly quicker, so it's highly recommended that you get this book, especially while it's free!

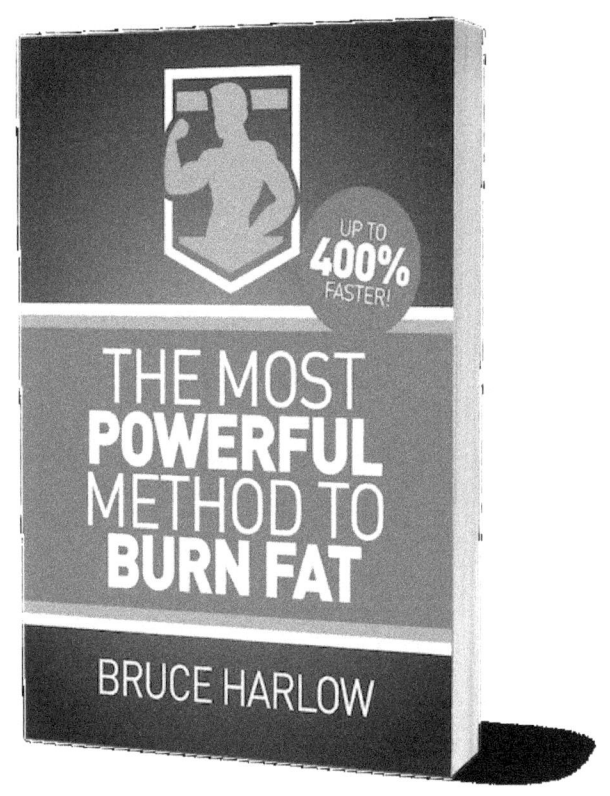

Get Your FREE Copy Here:

TopFitnessAdvice.com/Download

Chapter 1

Basic Principles of Weight Training

Weight training is one of the most common exercise programs used to develop physical fitness. Yet not everyone benefits from it the same way.

In these exercises, the muscles work to counteract the force exerted by gravity on weighted objects, such as barbells, dumbbells, or weight stacks. Let's take a closer look at how this works. When it came to weight training, "skeletal muscle" is a term that we made us of. In your body, there are three different categories of muscle tissue: smooth, cardiac, and skeletal. Every one of these is distinct in terms of what it does and its structure.

It doesn't take a genius to work out that cardiac muscle is what gets the heart moving but what is the difference between the other two types.

Smooth much comes under the classification of muscles that are involuntary. You cannot consciously control smooth muscle in any way. These can be found in the lining of your internal organs, the circulatory system, and also in your reproductive and digestive systems.

Skeletal muscle moves bones and other structures. These muscle fibers occur in muscles which are attached to the skeleton. These are muscles that you do have control over and muscles that have a striated appearance.

For this reason, weight training is targeting only the skeletal muscles.

However, there are also peripheral benefits to the cardiac muscles which will be discussed later in this book. There are other forms of exercises, however, that are more targeted towards the development of the cardiac muscle abilities.

The Overload and Progression Principle

In the world of sports science, overload and progression are two basic training principles that are often used as the basis for formulating an exercise program.

The human body is capable of making automatic adjustments to allow itself to be fit for survival.

When you suffer an injury, for example, the body does a complex system of bodily functions to repair the injured body part and make it stronger and more capable of resisting the injury the next time around.

The principle of overload tells us that a greater than usual stress or workload on the body is required for positive adaptation to take place.

The body will adapt to the stress stimulus by making the muscle stronger and bigger, depending on the type of load that it went through.

Once the body has adapted completely to the stimulus, then a different stimulus is required to continue to see change. This necessity to vary the amount of stimulus in order to continue to see change is the principle of progression.

Remember the old adage, "No pain, no gain."?

When we stress our muscles at a state above what they are used to, tears start to appear in them. (You have to use a microscope to see them.) This is a good thing, but the bigger the tear is, the more you are likely to be sore once you have finished training.

That's why it's important to advance more slowly. If you do this properly, your muscles will go into a hypertrophic state. In laymen's terms, this means that they'll increase the size to match the new "load" the body thinks you need to carry.

Unfortunately, some think that going full-speed ahead here is going to have the optimal effect. After all, what's a little muscle soreness?

The problem with thinking this way is that you could end up doing a lot of damage to your muscles and injure yourself. This will set you back in your program while you heal so work out a good compromise between intensity and protecting yourself from injuries.

There are essentially three ways in which you can increase the amount of workload to achieve the overload and progression necessary for muscle development:

1. Increase your training frequency
2. Increase your training duration
3. Increase your training intensity

The first two are self-explanatory. Increasing training intensity can be done in a variety of ways. You can increase training intensity through the following:

1. Increase the number of weights
2. Decrease the amount of rest between sets
3. Increase the repetition
4. Or any two or more combination of the above

How to Tell When Enough is Enough

One of the oldest ways to ensure that you are training enough is to train to failure. What this means is that you keep exercising until you are physically unable to do another rep without the help of your training partner or rest.

This is old science. Of, course this is proven to work. But we do not simply train to failure on each and every set. This book will guide you when to train to failure and when not to, for optimal growth and development.

There's a reason why the principle of overload and progression is the first order of business in this book. Almost all discussions about muscle development rely on these two building blocks of weight training knowledge.

If you do not train enough, the result is underdevelopment or no development at all. You will just be wasting your time. On the other hand, if you train too much, the results may be even more serious than before you even started, and you might suffer injury after injury.

Remember, the only way to truly achieve a genuine and lasting development in your physical fitness is to do the right training at the right amounts and at the right time.

How can we tell when enough is enough? When you have reached your target repetition or weight for an exercise, then that is enough. If you can do more than the prescribed reps, then you have got to load more weights.

There are specific exercises with a predefined target repetition. You have to stick to these targets. There are also exercises with target repetition that is set to "until failure." Then failure is the target (sounds weird, right?)

How do you set the right target? You'll find out in just a bit.

Chapter 2

Elements of an Effective Weight Training Program

The key to an effective weight training program are form, FITT, variety, and consistency.

Form

Probably the most important element of an effective workout is performing the exercises with the correct form. It is essential to ensuring that you get the most out of the exercise and helps avoid unnecessary injuries.

If you make a conscious effort to do things correctly especially in the early stages, your body will get used to the proper form that it will be almost automatic for your body to tell when you are exercising incorrectly.

This is what makes for **"instinctive training"** done by advanced athletes. If you are a beginner, focus on form more than anything else.

Until you have perfected the execution of an exercise in its correct, you should not move to heavier weights.

Otherwise, the errors in your execution will simply be magnified. Never sacrifice form for anything else.

The FITT Model

FITT is an acronym for Frequency, Intensity, Time, and Type. It is used as mnemonics to help you plan your fitness program, keeping in mind these four elements.

- **Frequency**

    This relates to the number of times that you perform an exercise program within a given period of time.

- **Intensity**

    Intensity relates to the amount of exertion that should be invested in a workout. As discussed in the previous chapter, you can vary the intensity by adjusting the amount of weights, repetition, rest between sets, or a combination of any of the three.

- **Time**

    The amount of time you spent on the workout is critical in determining whether your workout session makes a positive impact on your body.

    If the body is put into training for just the right amount of time, the nervous system releases growth hormones necessary for repair and development of the muscles. The time you spend on your workout will depend on your exercise program, which is determined by your set goals; more of this in the next chapter.

- **Type**

    An effective workout routine will normally include a variety of exercise types. Exercise types include lifting weights, doing isometric exercises, working on cardio exercises, among others.

    There's a wide variety of exercise types available, and you will need to incorporate a mix of these as you progress from beginner to advanced level in your weight training program.

- **Variety**

    An emphasis on variety helps create an impactful exercise program. The only way to make the muscles respond positively to stress is to continue to "shock" the muscles in ways that it does not normally expect. Monotony stunts growth and will create boredom in the long run. You need to have fun after all!

- **Consistency**

    Finally, what good would it do you if you have the ultimate workout but does not have the consistency to keep it going?

    Weight training is a discipline. If you fall into dormancy, you will lose whatever you have earned and worked so hard for.

Throughout the planning, execution, and evaluation periods of your weight training program, you need to keep all these key elements in mind. Some coaches only preach the FITT model, because it's easy to remember. But there are also other things. Form, variety, and consistency are a few other critical factors to take into consideration.

I hope that you are enjoying this book so far, and if you could spare 30 seconds, I would greatly appreciate you leaving a review on Amazon.com.

Chapter 3

Setting Your Goals

The importance of goal-setting before engaging in a weight training program cannot be overemphasized. Your goals determine what kind of workout program you will be creating.

It is going to be your basis for fitting the FITT model into your plan. First, you must decide if you are training to enhance your appearance, your physical performance, or both.

Training for Appearance

I am sure you will agree with me when I say that majority of the beginners in weight training wanted to train for appearance. They wanted to look leaner or bigger.

Either way, we need first to take a look at the status quo – what your body looks like now. Then we can determine what your specific goals are and how you are going to get there.

Understand Your Body Type

Your body type is initially determined by your genetic make-up – what you were born to look like. It's your original design. But with a constant and effective training program, you can actually change the way your body looks like.

The famous Arnold Schwarzenegger was born slender (ectomorph) when he started. His legs and calves were thin. He weighed a mere 150 lbs. at a height of 6'2". With sheer hard work and persistence, he eventually became a mesomorph and then went on to become the most decorated bodybuilder of his era.

George St. Pierre, considered one of the greatest UFC athletes ever, was born endomorph. Through a scientific approach to training and nutrition, he was able to transform his body into a lean athlete.

Here's what you need to learn about your body type.

1. **Ectomorph** – If you fall into this category, you have a delicate build and are naturally lean. Building muscle means more work for you but, if you are persistent, you can get it right.

   Over the course of later chapters, we will look at what the best workout for your body shape is and how it will differ from that of someone with a different body shape. Ectomorphs generally have:

   - Joints that are small in size
   - Lean appearance
   - Metabolism that seems to be on overdrive
   - Hyperactivity
   - The ability to eat anything without gaining weight
   - Satisfied with smaller portions
   - A smaller butt and chest
   - Trouble with gaining extra pounds
   - Finds it hard to build muscle
   - Narrow shoulders and hips

2. **Mesomorph** – In this instance, the frame is a little bigger, with their hips not being as wide as their shoulders. In a woman, this tends to create a nice hourglass figure.

   People who fall into this category are often strong, athletic, lean and compact. This is a great body shape to have as building muscle is easy to do. You might be a mesomorph if:

   - You build is symmetrical
   - Your hips are not as wide as your shoulders
   - You have a well-defined waist
   - You have a lower percentage of body fat
   - You have large muscles
   - You are able to add more muscle without a lot of effort.
   - It seems like you can easily burn off fat.
   - If you eat a reasonable amount of food.

3. **Endomorph** – This body shape is completely different to either mentioned before. Endomorphs tend to have a rounder body shape and carry a lot of fat. If most of the characteristics listed below apply to you, you can count yourself an endomorph:

   - A lot of fat on the body
   - Fatigued very easily, even with just a little exercise
   - Appetite can be voracious
   - Several attempts and dieting and exercising that ultimately failed
   - It is difficult to lose weight

- May be prone to snacking throughout the day or eating larger meals
- Muscles are not well defined and may be covered by a layer of fat
- Eat larger meals or several smaller sized meals
- Have a frame that is larger

Note that not everyone is a perfect ectomorph, endomorph, or mesomorph. In fact, only a few people are. Our body types belong to a spectrum, and people are normally somewhere in between.

For example, you may be born ecto-mesomorph or an endo-mesomorph. The level of mixture of your ecto/endo and meso qualities would also vary from others. You have to determine which one is your most dominant body type and in which part of the body type spectrum you belong to, so you can fit in your training accordingly.

Now that you have determined your body type, it's time to determine what kind of training you will undergo. Since this section talks about training for appearance, there is a couple of weight training programs we can use– body building and weight reduction

Bodybuilding

Bodybuilding is a sport, a discipline. But whether you train to become a bodybuilder or not, you can certainly use bodybuilding principles to enhance your appearance. The goal of bodybuilding is to develop the size of the muscles in such a way as to achieve a perfect combination of size and proportion while trimming down fat to as low as possible, to enhance muscle definition.

Aesthetics is hence the end-goal of bodybuilding, not strength, not power. If you are training for strength or power or endurance, bodybuilding may be supplemental but will not be the foundation for your training program.

If you are training to look bigger, or leaner, then bodybuilding is your tool. What is important at this stage is for you to decide whether to go this route or somewhere else.

Weight Reduction/Weight Loss Program

There are a variety of physical fitness programs available for weight loss. Weight training should be used in conjunction with other weight loss programs such as running, biking, or engaging on a certain sport. Weight training alone may also help achieve weight loss if you train the right way.

Training for Performance

Bodybuilding and weight training for weight loss are programs that will help you enhance appearance. But if your goal is to enhance your sports-specific physical abilities such as strength, speed, endurance, or power, then there are other forms of the program you should involve yourself in. Bodybuilding does not optimize strength. It aims to maximize lean muscle mass and eliminate fat.

Weight loss programs may improve your cardiovascular capacity, but if you are training for power, it will be difficult to achieve weight loss as loss of weight may put you at risk of losing power, especially if you are training to compete. Let us then distinguish between training for strength, endurance, and power.

Training for Strength

Weight training is best known for increasing strength. But the word strength can take varying definitions in daily language use.

Some will measure how heavy you lift, some will look at how many reps you take, or some will look at how far you can throw an object, how high you can jump, or how fast you can run. All of these abilities are different, yet they all connote strength. So, let's define here what we mean exactly by strength, at least in our context.

The sports definition of strength is the ability to carry out work against resistance. In order to increase muscle strength, your training program should include weight-lifting or some sort of resistance exercise.

So, for our use in this weight training book, we will measure strength based on how much you lift. If I can lift 100 lbs. of bench press in 8 reps and you can lift 75 lbs. in 20 reps, I am stronger than you, based on our definition. If I can bench press a maximum of 150 lbs. With only one full repetition and cannot do another one, then my one-rep max is 150 lbs. We will use one-rep max in this book to measure your strength in a particular exercise.

Evaluate your personal weight training goal to see if you want to train for strength only or a combination of strength and other elements of your physical performance. Powerlifters train for strength. Their one-rep max in bench press, squats, and deadlifts are the measures of their performance.

Bodybuilders do not train for strength. Although strength is a side-effect of their training, their ultimate goal is the perfection of mass, shape, and definition of the muscles.

Training for Power

In sports, power is defined as the person's ability for exertion over the shortest possible time. (So, things like sprinting, throwing a javelin and running a course of hurdles, require power.)

This is different to strength in that the time factor is more of a play for power.

Power is attributed to an explosive burst of movements. It is what weightlifters need. Strangely enough, powerlifters train more for strength than for power, because you do not need to be very explosive in the lifts that you do in powerlifting.

But, note that since power is strength x speed, you cannot achieve power unless you have strength.

If you are training for the high jump, long jump, a throwing event, weightlifting, arm wrestling, or combat sports like boxing, power is your key to victory. Sprinters also need power (remember that power is strength x speed). You need to decide if this is the route you will take.

Training for Endurance

Endurance is usually associated with cardiovascular endurance. But we can also use it for skeletal muscle endurance and define it as the ability to exercise continuously for extended periods without tiring.

If we can both lift 100 lbs. in barbell curls but I can only do 10 reps, and you can do 20 reps with the same amount of weight, then you muscle endurance at the 100-lb lift is better than mine. It may, of course, vary when we change the amount of weight being lifted, or when we alter the exercise.

The aerobic capacity or cardiovascular endurance that someone has refers to how efficient the system is when it comes to delivering oxygen to where it is needed most. (In our case, this will be to the muscles.)

The better your aerobic capacity is, the longer you are able to carry on exercising for. Endurance, in this respect, can be improved through the use of weight training and your normal cardiovascular training.

Endurance is needed by medium- and long-distance runners, swimmers, ball players, and many other athletes who have to deal with long periods of activity.

Understanding your Current Level of Performance

Every athlete or fitness enthusiast have varying levels of capacity and abilities, which is mostly dependent on their experience, amount of time spent on their specific sport or discipline, and their innate talents.

We categorize levels into 3: beginner, intermediate, and advanced. A 4th level, the elite level is where the outliers of sports and fitness are.

When you reach that level, you would already know what to do and would probably be able to design your own program based on what works for you and what doesn't. At this point, you need to determine which level you're at, so you can tailor your fitness program based on your current level.

Each fitness level has a different degree of difficulty so that you can progress a stage at a time to reach your goals. To know where in the program you should start, you need to establish your own personal baseline.

Don't let "helpful" advice about you ought to do or what you are able to do get you down. Each of us is built differently and have strengths that we can draw on. There is scope for improvement at each level of this program.

Don't be put off if you do fall into the category of beginners – you know your body and what it can do. Ignoring that could lead to disaster.

Here's what each category means and what types of exercises you will want to include:

- **Beginners**: This is someone who has not been working out regularly. Someone who may be new to working out at all. You need to start off slowly. Look at exercises that help build muscle memory and strength. Make sure you are using the right form here.

    As a beginner, you will start off with exercises designed to be easier to execute and performed at low intensity. You should spend less time working out to start off with and have little variety in the exercises that you do.

    You might want to get onto something a little more challenging, but these exercises provide the perfect base for your advancement to the next level.

- **Intermediates**: If you have been working out for quite a while and are now able to perform more advanced exercises, the Intermediate stage is more challenging and builds on what you have learned already.

    If you fall into this category, you will know how you should stand, etc. when exercising. Exercising in this category is more intense and longer.

- **Advanced**: These are people who are used to pushing their bodies to get the best out of them. They work on building speed, power, intensity, and strength so that they get extraordinary results. It will get to a stage where it becomes more difficult to start seeing improvements.

Be honest here, which category do you really belong in? If you want the best possible results, you need to face facts about your own levels of fitness or risk being disappointed.

Chapter 4

Safety First

I know you are excited to get started with your weight training program. But before you 'break a leg' and make a literal meaning out of it instead of figurative, let's get to a couple more basic but very important part of your training -the warm-up and the cool-down, the alpha and the omega of your workouts.

Warm-up

From beginner to elite athletes, no one is exempt to warm-ups. Everyone needs it and does it. Warming up helps to slowly gear your cardiovascular system up by heating your body and increasing the circulation of blood. Your muscles get more of the nutrients that they need, and you will be less prone to stiffness in the morning or injuring yourself.

Here is where it gets a little tricky. How much warm-up is necessary? The answer depends on your workout program. Keep in mind that too much warm-up will have a negative effect on the overall effectiveness of your workout?

For example, if you are planning to lift your one rep max in your workout and tired up your muscles even before your first one-rep max attempt, you will have set yourself up for failure. You may not be able to lift or exceed the one-rep max that you aimed for because you have already used up your muscle and some amount of fatigue has settled in.

In contrast, not enough warm-ups may lead to injury when your joints are not lubricated enough or may cause heart problems in the long-term when your heart is regularly subjected to sudden heavy loads.

Since warm-up is such a critical part of your workout, I will give a few hacks on how to do warm-ups. First, we need to find out your one-rep max (1RM).

One-Rep Max

Finding out your 1RM for a specific exercise is not part of your warm up nor your regular routine. You find this out separately.

These formulas will help you work out your 1RM:
Start with the upper body. What weights can you lift 4-6 times before being exhausted? Take the heaviest and use it here:

(4-6RM X 1.1307) + 0.6998.

So, let's say that the heaviest of these weights is 40kg, your formula would look something like:

(40 x 1.1307) + 0.6998.

Your IRM, in this case, would be 45.93 kg or 46kg.

You work out your 1RM for the lower body in the same way. The formula is a little different, though,

(4-6RM x 1.09703) + 14.2546.

If you want an easier way, you also check out different websites that provide a free 1RM calculator. You will have a different 1RM for every exercise. You need to record this information regularly to determine the amount you will lift on a certain day and whether you can start to progress or not.

Let's say that you decide to build some muscle through lifting, and you decide that you will do three sets with ten reps in each, you know that you ought to train at around three quarters of your 1RM.

If you do this, you should be able to finish all the sets at the best weight possible for muscle-building.

This makes your workouts a whole lot more effective. You will no longer set too low a weight and miss out on building your muscles. By the same token, you would also never overdo it either. It is the smart way to train.

As you progress, you will need to do this test again. How often this is will be completely determined by what you aim to achieve. A powerlifter, for example, is going to have very different goals to a bodybuilder, for example.

With the former, the 1RM plays a big part in you achieving your goal and so should be tested more often, maybe on a quarterly or bi-monthly basis.

A bodybuilder, on the other, is able to monitor progress by seeing the visual difference in their body and so may be able to get away with just once or twice year.

Stretching

We grew up being told that you had to stretch before you exercised to reduce the chances of injuring yourself.

Now, however, research seems to indicate that static stretching as a warm-up is not going to reduce the risk of injuring yourself or even help you perform better.

Having said that, it's also not going to be bad for you either. Bouncing, PNF and dynamic stretches have been proven to have greater efficacy rates.

Below are the types of stretching:

- **Static stretch**: Here you hold stretch out the muscle until you feel a slight pull. You then stay in the position for at least 30 seconds.

- **Proprioceptive neuromuscular facilitation (PNF)**: There are a lot of different techniques used to get this right, but you are basically stretching out the muscle and then alternately relaxing and contracting it.

- **Dynamic stretch**: In this case, you repeat gentle movements over and over again. Like swinging your arms, for example. What makes this a stretch is that you continue to change the range of motion. (But always stay within normal limits.)

- **Bouncing or Ballistic stretches**: In this case, you stretch the muscle and then bounce or jerk it to help deepen the stretch.

The sure thing about stretching is it prepares the muscle for bigger work. Stretching works the muscle. However, you have to be careful not to commit a common mistake – stretching a cold muscle.

Stretching a Cold Muscle

This may sound crazy – we are told to stretch before a workout. Won't the muscles be cold anyway? Never stretch your muscles when they are cold, or you could be impeding your progress.

What I mean by this is that you start off your session with static stretches.

Let's look at what happens when you do this – the stretch makes your muscle fibers lengthen temporarily. If the muscles are completely cold, they haven't got the increased blood flow into them that exercise would bring yet, and this makes them prone to tearing.

Take two elastic bands, for example – one hot and one warm. Which one will stretch more easily? Which one will be more brittle and prone to break? If you do stretch the cold one out, how easy will it be for it to get back into shape again?

Static stretching as a warm-up is likely to do more harm than good. Rather start with a light cardio workout for around five minutes. Jog on the spot, walk to the gym, etc. – anything that gets the blood pumping.

This will increase blood-flow to your muscles and also increase your body temperature, allowing your body to warm up naturally.

If you do want to stretch during your warm-up, dynamic stretching is the way to go. This involves actively moving your body using rolls, kicks, and swings. These help to loosen up the joints and improve your range of motion. It can help to keep the joints flexible.

And, because you are only working on a particular area, the blood-flow is increased to that area, making it easier to warm up. As long as you remember the golden rule – stretch until you feel a little discomfort. Pain is not gain in this case at all. Some examples of this kind of stretching are circling your arms, kicking your legs and rolling your hips.

Fitness Hack: Warm-up

Here's a sample warm-up hack routine that you can use in any strength-building and power-building exercise. Remember that your goal is only to warm your muscles, not tire them. Your muscle's maximum capacity should not be decreased in any way during the warm-up.

1. At the start of the workout session, do 5-10 minutes of moderate exercise – walking, cycling, jogging or other forms of light cardiovascular activity.

2. Start each exercise with 8-12 reps of 50% 1RM. For example, you will do 5 sets of bench press. You need to do your first set with 8-12 reps of 50% 1RM.

3. Do light stretching for a minute (dynamic stretch)

4. Proceed with slightly heavier second set (70% of your 1RM in 8-10 reps)

This completes the warm up for that exercise. Note that step 1 is a warm up for the whole day's session while step 2 to 4 is a warm-up to be done for each exercise that has at least 5 sets.

This sets up your muscle for the greater load and fun ahead. For an exercise with only 3 sets required, you can skip these warm up sets.

Cool-Down

Cooling down after you work out lets your body recover naturally. It can help to slow down your heart rate and the rate at which you were breathing to a slow and steady pace.

This helps to prevent dizziness or fainting. It also prevents the blood from pooling in the large muscles when you stop and will assist in the removal of waste buildup, like lactic acid.

Cooling down is as simple as warming up. Jog or walk for about five minutes to help reduce your temperature and speed waste away from the muscles. Follow with about five minutes of static stretching to complete the process.

Once again, thank you for reading this book, and I hope you're getting a lot of valuable information. I would greatly appreciate it if you could take 30 seconds to leave me a review for this book on Amazon.com.

Enjoying this book?

Check out our other best sellers!

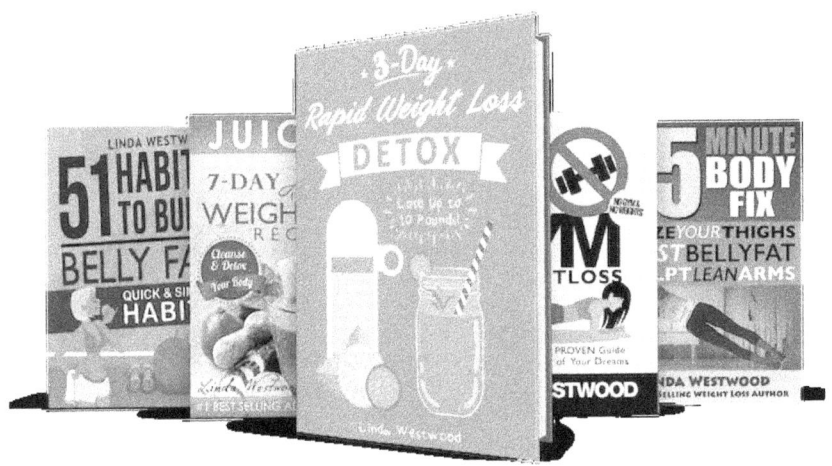

Get your next book on sale here:

TopFitnessAdvice.com/go/books

Chapter 5

Killer Weight Training Programs Part 1: Training for Appearance

You've set your goal; you've done your warm-up; now it is time to get your hands on the iron. I will show you fitness hacks and sample workout programs that you can mimic or modify depending on your level of fitness and what you find to work best for you.

It is important that you have set your goals before reaching this section in order for you to avoid wasting time. If you have not done this yet, go back to Chapter 3.

Fitness Hack: Weight Training Part 1

The first thing we'll look at is bodybuilding. Here are key fitness hacks you have to remember:

1. **Combine isolation exercises with compound exercises.**

    The most common way to improve a muscle is to isolate them. Bicep curls isolate the biceps. The bench press isolates the chest but also works the triceps and shoulders to some extent.

    The best way to grow your muscles is to do a combination of compound and isolation exercises. Doing compound exercises such as squats, deadlift, and pull-ups help trigger your nervous system to release growth hormones, compared to just focusing on isolation exercises.

2. **Strive for optimal intensity.**

This doesn't mean you have to lift your 1RM all the time. No. But you have to continue to challenge your muscles to develop beyond its current levels. This is the only way for a workout to become effective – you have to find ways to shock the muscles.

In bodybuilding, it is important to focus on both the amount of weight and the number of repetitions. This will increase muscle mass while ensuring that body fat is minimized. Bodybuilding repetition is 6 to 12 reps, with decreasing reps in succeeding sets. For example, set 1 is 12 reps, set 2 is 10, set 3 is 8, set 4 is 8 and set 5 is 6.

3. **Rest each body part for 4 days.**

This might appear counter-intuitive to you, especially for those who have been bodybuilding for a while now. But have you noticed that your lifts aren't improving as much? And there are days you just feel weak or too tired to workout. That's because your muscles aren't getting enough rest.

Remember that the only way for muscles to grow is when you rest and nourish them properly after an intense and effective workout that shocks your muscles. You will see how this rest period works out in a sample program later. The idea is simple: **Work hard, rest hard.**

4. **Breathing**

   Exhale during the exertion phase of the movement. Inhale during the negative phase of the movement.

   For example, when doing squats, you inhale as much oxygen as possible while going down (negative phase). On your way up (exertion phase), slowly release your breath in a smooth rhythm. One technique to ensure you are able to do this: count out loud during each exertion phase movement to make sure you are exhaling. "One, two, and three..."

5. **Spotters**

   A spotter is a person who assists lifter during an exercise movement in order to minimize the chance of accidents or injuries and to help finish out a movement. A spot is defined as **"absolute minimum assistance."**

   The spotters should not be lifting any more than you do. They should be exerting very minimal assistance. If you see a spotter struggling, it's a signal that you are lifting too much for your own good. You need to reduce the amount of weight.

   Nevertheless, spotters are useful in your workout. However, you should not be calling spotters unless it's your last 1-2 sets of a particular exercise. For example, if you are doing 5 sets of military press, you shouldn't need a spotter to help you on sets 1 to 3.

On set 4 or 5, the spotter will be able to help you squeeze out the last 2 to 4 reps, but you should be able to make at least 2 reps on your own.

It is the final 1 or 2 reps in your exercise that shocks your muscle because by this time your muscles have already reached a point of failure or overload, lifting more than it can normally take.

Having a spotter to assist you to finish the movement enables the body to recruit all possible muscle fibers that it can recruit at that moment, causing the maximum effect that will stimulate muscle hypertrophy (muscle growth).

6. Ketosis

In its simplest terms, ketosis is a process during which fat is converted to ketones — a perfectly usable energy source for every major body system. The body, though, has a limit to how much fat it burns.

After it reaches this threshold, it turns to other fuel sources, particularly protein. And you do not want to burn your protein which you want to use for muscle growth.

Thus, if you are gaining weight, you have to keep the fat burning process only up to the point that it does not have to turn to protein next.

Even if your goal is to lose weight, doing more cardiovascular exercise than you are supposed to do does not burn that extra fat, it only depletes your body of glycogen and protein in the liver and muscles.

Weight Gain vs. Weight Loss

Now let's apply these few principles into a sample workout routine for bodybuilding. Remember that your bodybuilding program will depend on your body type and your fitness goal. We will show two types of programs, weight gain, and weight reduction.

Weight Gain

Note that the repetitions stated here are in minimum. If you can squeeze more, do so, but make sure to record it accordingly. If you can do more reps than recommended it means you can increase the amount of weight.

If you are unable to accomplish the recommended reps at the recommended weight, either get a spotter or reduce the amount of weight. Review the previous section discussing spotters to discern which action to take.

The program is set to 5 days. If you start Day 1 on a Monday, you will finish the first week on Friday, and then start your new Day 1 on Saturday. One advantage of this is it reduces monotony in your routine.

So, you can't say Monday is always leg day, some weeks it will be chest day or even rest day. But the main principle is to ensure you have a 4-day rest period. Your Day 4 is dedicated to weak point training. You can choose which body you want to train twice a weak.

For example, if your calves are very small and recover pretty fast even when you need a 4-day rest, you can choose calves to be trained on Day 4.

Note that this is also your cardio day. You will spend 30 minutes to an hour of running, biking, swimming or playing sports, whatever will work-out your cardiovascular endurance. Make sure to limit this to no more than an hour since this is a weight gain program, and any excess may lead to weight loss which is opposite of what you want to achieve.

Follow this program and expect to see results in less than a month!

Schedule	Body Part	Exercise	# of Sets	# of Repetition	Remarks
		Program 1A (weight gain for beginners)			
Day 1	Legs	Barbell Squat	5	12,10,9,8,6,6	Includes 2 warm-up sets
		Hamstring Curls	3	12,10,8	
		Leg Press	3	12,10,8	
		Leg Extensions	3	12,10,8	
	Biceps	Barbell Curls	5	12,10,9,8,6,6	
		Seated incline dumbbell curls	3	12,10,8	
	Abs	Crunch	5	50	
		Reverse Crunch	5	50	
Day 2	Chest	Barbell Bench Press	5	12,10,9,8,6,6	
		Incline Dumbbell Press	4	10,9,8,7	
		Dumbbell Flys	3	12,10,8	
	Triceps	Dips- Triceps Version	5	8 to 12	
		Dumbbell One-Arm Triceps Extension	3	10,9,8	
	Calves	Standing Calf Raises	6	25-30	
	Abs	Knee Raises	5	50	
		Oblique Crunch	5	50	
Day 3	Back	Chin-ups	Unlimited	total of 50	can be replaced by cable pull-ups to adjust the weights if you are unable to do 50 reps of chin-ups
		Bent Over Barbell Row	4	10,9,8,7	
		Seated Cable Row	3	12,10,8	
	Shoulders	Clean and Press	4	10,9,8,7	
		Standing Military Press	4	10,9,8,7	
		Side Lateral Raise	4	10,9,8,7	
	Abs	Crunch	5	50	
		Reverse Crunch	5	50	
Day 4		Weakpoint training		Pick only one weak point. You can also vary your choice every week.	
		Cardio Day			
Day 5		Rest			

Weight Loss

The program for weight loss is not much different from the weight gain except for the repetition and volume of the workout. You can slightly modify the number of reps and sets, but these are the minimum.

Or you can stick to the prescribed amount of reps and sets and increase the weights instead. I prefer the latter as this assures your muscles get the maximum benefit from weight training.

You should not exceed more than 12 reps on most of the lifting exercises even if you are doing weight loss program because doing so will not be beneficial to your strength development.

If you are able to build quality muscle (which comes from increased muscle strength), then these muscles are going to be the ones burning the fat under your skin by improving your basal metabolic rate, which is the rate at which your body burns calories even when you are doing nothing.

The bigger the muscles, the more calories it needs to burn to simply maintain itself.

So, in weight training, though the weight loss program will have slightly more reps and sets than the weight gain program, the goal is still to build the strength and size of the muscles. The increased rep and sets will have a positive effect on endurance.

Program 2A (weight loss for beginners)

Schedule	Body Part	Exercise	# of Sets	# of Repetition	Remarks
Day 1	Legs	Barbell Squat	5	12,10,9,8,8,8	includes 2 warm-up sets
		Hamstring Curls	5	12,10,9,8,8,8	
		Leg Press	5	12,10,9,8,8,8	
		Leg Extensions	3	12,10,8	
	Biceps	Barbell Curls	5	12,10,9,8,8,8	
		Seated incline dumbbell curls	5	12,10,9,8,8,8	
	Abs	Crunch	5	failure	minimum of 50
		Reverse Crunch	5	failure	minimum of 50
Day 2	Chest	Barbell Bench Press	5	12,10,9,8,8,8	
		Incline Dumbbell Press	4	12,10,8,8	
		Dumbbell Flys	3	12,10,8	
	Triceps	Dips- Triceps Version	5	8 to 12	
		Dumbbell One-Arm Triceps Extension	3	12,10,8	
	Calves	Standing Calf Raises	6	25-30	
	Abs	Knee Raises	5	failure	minimum of 50
		Oblique Crunch	5	failure	minimum of 50
Day 3	Back	Chin-ups	Unlimited	total of 50	can be replaced by cable pull-ups to adjust the weights if you are unable to do 50 reps of chin-ups
		Bent Over Barbell Row	4	12,10,8,8	
		Seated Cable Row	3	12,10,8	
	Shoulders	Clean and Press	4	12,10,8,8	
		Standing Military Press	4	12,10,8,8	
		Side Lateral Raise	4	12,10,8,8	
	Abs	Crunch	5	failure	minimum of 50
		Reverse Crunch	5	failure	minimum of 50
Day 4		Weakpoint training		Pick only one weak point. You can also vary your choice every week.	
		Cardio Day			
Day 5		Rest			

Intermediate Level

After spending 1 to 2 months on the beginner level, you should have made some significant progress in your strength and endurance and is now ready to move on to intermediate level. The maximum you can stay in the beginner's stage is three months.

Therefore, it is imperative to leave procrastination behind and keep your progress in check. Do not stay at the beginner level for more than three months or you will notice that there is no progress to be found.

You will have plateaued already by that time, and since the routine becomes "normal" for the muscles, it no longer finds a trigger for growth and development.

The amount of progress you will have attained after completing the beginner depends on the amount of work that you have put in and the consistency. Rest and nutrition are also just as important as your workout. Here's a hack – **before moving on to the next level, take a full week off.**

Here's why: your body needs time off to fully recuperate from the continuous workout. It needs a semi-off season. After the full week when you get back to training your body will be shocked again and growth and development, which may have stopped already due to some kid of initial plateau, will be triggered again. Remember the shock principle?

At the intermediate level, we introduce you to some new set of exercises to add to your routine – the power exercises. In the beginner level, you only had the clean and press as your power exercise. This should have conditioned your nervous system to do more of the same nature of exercises.

Some additional power exercises we will add are the push presses, deadlift, and the snatch. We will also add half squats, maxi-isolation of the biceps, and other exercises that will force your muscles to lift heavier weights and continue to develop.

Below are sample workouts for both weight loss and weight gain. The difference in the amount of sets and reps between the two programs narrows as we reach the intermediate level, where both individuals will be about close to their goals by now, if not at it. Can you spot the difference?

Program 1B (weight gain for intermediate level)

Schedule	Body Part	Exercise	# of Sets	# Reps per Set	Remarks
Day 1	Legs	Barbell Squat	3	10,8,6	
		Half-Squats	2	8,6	Very Heavy weights
		Hamstring Curls	3	10,8,6	
		Leg Press	3	10,8,6	
		Dumbbell Lunge	3	10,8,6	
	Biceps	Barbell Curls	4	10,8,6,6	
		Single arm bench bicep curls	2	8,6	very heavy weights
		Dumbbell-Alternate-Bicep-Curl-With-Twist	2	8,6	
	Abs	Continuous crunches 25 reps each: Crunch, Reverse Crunch, Leg Raises, Bicycle	5	total of 100 reps per set	
Day 2	Chest	Barbell Bench Press	4	10,8,6,6	
		Half Bench Press	2	8,6	
		Incline Dumbbell Press	3	12,10,8	
		Standing Cable Flys	3	12,10,8	
	Shoulders	Clean and Press	4	10,9,8,7	
		Push Press	2	8,6	
		Snatch	3	8,8,6	
		Arnold Dumbbell Press	3	10,8,8	
	Abs	Vertical Leg Raise	5	25	
		Plank	3	-	each set to failure
Day 3	Back	Chin-ups	5	at least 10 or to failure	
		Deadlift	3	8,6,6	
		Single Arm Dumbbell Row	3	10,8,8	
	Triceps	Cable Tricep Pushdown	4	10,8,6,6	
		Incline EZ bar lying tricep extension	3	10,9,8	
	Calves	Standing Calf Raises	4	25-30	
		Seated Claf Raise	4	25-30	
	Abs	Decline Reverse Crunch	5	25	
		Ab Wheel Rollout	5	25	
Day 4		Weakpoint training		Pick only one weak point. You can also vary your choice every week.	
		Cardio Day			
Day 5		Rest			

Program 2B (weight loss for intermediate level)

Schedule	Body Part	Exercise	# of Sets	# Reps per Set	Remarks
Day 1	Legs	Barbell Squat	5	10,8,6	
		Half-Squats	2	8,6	Very Heavy weights
		Hamstring Curls	4	10,8,6	
		Leg Press	3	10,8,6	
		Dumbbell Lunge	3	10,8,6	
	Biceps	Barbell Curls	4	10,8,6,6	
		Single arm bench bicep curls	2	8,6	very heavy weights
		Dumbbell-Alternate-Bicep-Curl-With-Twist	2	8,6	
	Abs	Continuous crunches 25 reps each: Crunch, Reverse Crunch, Leg Raises, Bicycle	5	total of 100 reps per set	
Day 2	Chest	Barbell Bench Press	5	10,8,6,6	
		Half Bench Press	2	8,6	
		Incline Dumbbell Press	4	12,10,8	
		Standing Cable Flys	3	12,10,8	
	Shoulders	Clean and Press	4	10,9,8,7	
		Push Press	2	8,6	
		Snatch	3	8,8,6	
		Arnold Dumbbell Press	3	10,8,8	
	Abs	Vertical Leg Raise	5	25	
		Plank	3	-	each set to failure
Day 3	Back	Chin-ups	5	at least 10 or to failure	
		Deadlift	4	8,6,6	
		Single Arm Dumbbell Row	3	10,8,8	
	Triceps	Cable Tricep Pushdown	5	10,8,6,6	
		Incline EZ bar lying tricep extension	3	10,9,8	
	Calves	Standing Calf Raises	5	25-30	
		Seated Claf Raise	5	25-30	
	Abs	Decline Reverse Crunch	5	25	
		Ab Wheel Rollout	5	25	
Day 4		Weakpoint training		Pick only one weak point. You can also vary your choice every week.	
		Cardio Day			
Day 5		Rest			

You will notice that the program for abs workout has become quiet more interesting and diverse. Day 1 for ab workout includes a super combo in which each set consist of 100 continuous reps made up of 4 different exercises of 25 reps each.

We have also switched the schedules and combination of some body parts to maintain balance in total intensity for each day. You will also notice some of the exercises remain. These are the staple exercises its corresponding body parts.

Advanced Level

Before moving on to advanced level, you will need a full week of rest, away from training, just like you did when you moved from beginner to intermediate level.

In the advanced level, the focus is on additional volume and diversity. This is the time when you can experiment on new exercises and add several different flavors to your workout, in order to continue to shock your muscle to new levels.

For illustration purposes, I used some similar exercise in beginner and intermediate level to show how the number of sets and reps should look like. The total volume of work is important. It shouldn't be more nor less than adequate. More will result in overtraining while less will result in plateauing and lack of development.

Notice the difference in the number of exercises and the reps and sets between intermediate and advanced. From here you can either mimic the program or do something creative on your own. Mix and match! Remember that at this level, intensity, volume, and diversity is what matters the most.

Program 1C/2C (weight gain and weight loss advanced level)

Schedule	Body Part	Exercise	# of Sets	# Reps per Set	Remarks
Day 1	Legs	Barbell Squat	3	10,8,6	
		Half-Squats	2	8,6	Very Heavy weights
		Hamstring Curls	3	10,8,6	
		Single Leg Press	3	10,8,6	
		Leg Extension	3	10,8,6	
		Dumbbell Lunge	3	10,8,6	
	Biceps	Barbell Curls	3	10,8,6,6	
		Cheat curls	2	8,6	
		Single arm bench bicep curls	2	8,6	very heavy weights
		Dumbbell-Alternate-Bicep-Curl-With-Twist	2	8,6	
		Overhead Cable Curls	2	10,8	
	Abs	Continuous crunches 50 reps each: Crunch, Reverse Crunch, Leg Raises, Bicycle	5	total of 200 reps per set	
Day 2	Chest	Barbell Bench Press	4	10,8,6,6	
		Machine Chest Press	3	8,6	Very Heavy weights
		Incline Dumbbell Press	3	12,10,8	
		Incline Chest Flys	3	12,10,8	
	Shoulders	Clean and Press	4	10,9,8,7	
		Push Press	2	8,6	
		Snatch	3	8,8,6	
		Side Lateral Raise	3	10,8,8	
		Arnold Dumbbell Press	3	10,8,8	
	Abs	Vertical Leg Raise	5	50	
		Plank	3	-	each set to failure
Day 3	Back	Chin-ups	5	at least 10 or to failure	
		Deadlift	3	8,6,6	
		Single Arm Dumbbell Row	3	10,8,8	
		Seated Cable Row	3	12,10,8	
	Triceps	Cable Tricep Pushdown	4	10,8,6,6	
		Incline EZ bar lying tricep extension	3	10,9,8	
		Dumbbell One-Arm Triceps Extension	3	10,9,8	
	Calves	Standing Calf Raises	6	30-35	
		Seated Claf Raise	6	30-35	
	Abs	Decline Reverse Crunch	5	50	
		Ab Wheel Rollout	5	50	
Day 4		Weakpoint training			Pick only one weak point. You can also vary your choice every week.
		Cardio Day			
Day 5		Rest			

So far, we have discussed and illustrated sample programs that would help us achieve our goal – enhance our appearance. By the end of the intermediate level you should already be at your desired level and ready to advance further.

When you have been at the advanced level for at least a couple of months, you may or may not want to consider competing as well. It is all for you to decide. So, how do you look now?

Others who are considering purchasing this book would love to know what you think. If you could spare a few seconds, they would greatly appreciate reading an honest review from you. Simply visit the page on Amazon.com.

Chapter 6

Killer Weight Training Programs Part 2: Training for Performance

Other than training for appearance, we can also choose to focus on training for performance. Weight training can indeed help us achieve gains in strength, endurance, power, and speed, which we will need in our particular sport, or maybe just for the fun of it.

In the first one month of weight training, the physical improvements are pretty noticeable and significant. In the second and third month, the rate and amount of improvement you gain slowly decreases.

By the end of the 3rd month, you will need to put more than the normal amount of hard work to continue to shock your muscles beyond the plateau. Let me share with you a few fitness hacks and sample workout for improving beyond your first plateau point.

Fitness Hack: Weight Training Part 2

1. **Rest between Sets.** The amount of rest between your sets is a great determinant to the workout's intensity.

   To calculate your rest time when working out, consider the following guidelines:

Goal: Building endurance in muscles. Start with reps of 12 to 20 followed by a rest of 30 to 45 seconds.

Goal: Hypertrophy. Start with reps of 6 to 12 followed by a rest of 60 to 90 seconds.

Goal: Stronger muscles. Start with reps of 3 to 5 followed by a rest of 2 to 4 minutes.

Goal: More powerful muscles. Start with reps of 1 to 3 followed by a rest of 60 to 90 seconds.

2. **Forced Rep.** You can consider a rep "forced" if you achieve muscle failure while doing a set and have a partner help you complete the set. This takes you past your standard point of failure, and so has a greater impact on the muscles. This improves muscle density and growth.

3. **Forced Negatives.** These are when you repeatedly execute the lift's eccentric stage. So, as an example, if you are bench pressing, that negative move would be when you bring the bar down to the chest. The eccentric stage of the lift is when your muscle is lengthened.

Remember, the eccentric phase of a lift occurs when the muscle lengthens. In squats, bicep curls or bench presses, this is during the downward phase.

The opposite of this, the concentric stage, happens as the muscle starts to shorten, like when you extend your arms up when bench pressing. Forcing the negative stage means that you make use of weights that are very heavy and that you hold the negative stage for longer. It is a good idea to have someone spotting you when you do this.

Negatives help add higher intensity when working out and help to overload those muscles groups active during the exercise. You can include negatives by lowering the weight more slowly and slowing the temp to match. You should aim for a rep count of 3 to 5 seconds.

It becomes necessary to include these moves when you are no longer seeing any progress from your usual workouts. (Usually, that is when you feel sore enough to know you've had a productive workout.

There is a caveat here, though. These can strain your tendons and joints. If you are going to incorporate these often, be prepared for injuries due to overuse.

Because you are essentially using more weight than you are able to life, you will need to have someone helping you lift the weigh and then let go when you are lowering it.

4. **Partial Rep.** This is also known as a half-rep, and it makes use of a limited range of motion while mimicking the full range of motion. The old school wisdom is that we need to get a full range of motion in order to get the full benefit of an exercise.

But in this case, we will be increasing the weight on the limited-range-of-motion lift in order so that you get stronger when it comes to that full-range-of-motion lift.

It is not going to be your bread and butter but only supplemental to your training.

5. **One-Rep Set.** We mentioned this before – muscles that are strong will usually also be bigger and have more capacity to do work. Working at maximum when it comes to strength training helps to build up your skeletal structure and thicken the connective tissues. This helps to carry the new muscles and also prevents injury, now and as you age.

   The fastest, and best, way for you to get really strong is to start lifting the weights that are as heavy as possible. If you can do more than one rep, it is not heavy enough. You need a weight that you battle to lift. It may not sound like a lot of work, but it is extremely tiring. You will feel exhausted afterwards.

   It's a different kind of tired, though. You won't feel much of a burn in the muscles, but you are going to have to concentrate completely. The shorter sets and the increased period of rest between them do, however, make this a less hectic training schedule.

   And the results will speak for themselves.

6. **Cheat Reps.** This is a rep that is performed less strictly so that you can use weights that are a lot heavier. A great example here is your normal dumbbell curl, repeated until failure, and then followed with reps using body swing or knee-bends. You could also get the shoulders and legs to assist you if you are executing barbell rows.

There is a lot of controversy in fitness circles about these – some trainers won't allow them at all. That said, they do have benefits that have been proven time and time again.

They should, however, be a supplement to your normal routine, and not done throughout each set. You can leave them for the very last sets so that you can get the very last drop of strength out of the muscles and forcing them to build.

7. **Pulse Reps.** These are the variation on the theme of partial reps. They make use of a shorter movement range at about one or two inches only, when it comes to movement. This is paired by weights that are much heavier. Start off slowly, by using it to build up your biceps and see if you like the results. Then move on to the next body part.

8. **Superset.** These are when you execute a couple of different exercises in quick succession without much, if any, rest period between them. You would ordinarily do this body parts considered complementary to get the best effect. As an example, you could follow bench pressing with chin-ups. Or follow bicep curls with triceps extensions.

9. **Off-Season.** When it comes to weight training, consistency must be maintained to see good results. That said, you should not be training at maximum year-round. Your body needs some time off to recover fully and neglecting this could halt your progress for ages or even cause your condition to decline. Every year you will

need to take between one and two months off so that your body is able to restore itself completely.

That doesn't mean no training at all – your workouts during this time will be designed to grow muscles rather than increasing endurance. Here you will pay less attention to muscle fatigue, encouraging it to help build muscle mass. So, you would use lighter weights, so the workout is not as intense.

You could do around 3 to 5 sets of each chosen exercise. Each set would be around 10 to 15 reps, and you would aim to work out at no more than 75% intensity. Rest periods would be between 30 and 60 seconds between each set. If you are doing circuit training, as little rest as possible would be advised.

10. **Plyometrics.** Those wanting to improve power and strength often combine plyometrics and weight-training. This must be done with some thought, though if you want the maximum efficiency.

    If you aim to increase strength through weight lifting and increase explosive power through plyometrics, it is necessary to rest your muscles properly in between. It is during the rest days that your muscles do the most work – adapting, healing and recovering.

    You could combine the workouts if each is working a different set of muscles. So, weight lifting for your lower-body and plyometrics for the upper body.

This type of session should be held twice a week and with no more than four lots a week. As the volume and intensity are high, you must allow yourself two days rest between each workout.

So, you could do one combination on Mondays and Thursdays and the other on Wednesdays and Saturdays. Sunday would be a complete rest.

Do a good warm-up and make sure it is dynamic before starting out. This helps to warm the neuromuscular system which, in turn, reduces the chances of injuring yourself. Your warmup should be around 10 or 15 minutes long. Start off with a bit of light cardiovascular exercise to get going and then do dynamic stretching.

You can then move onto the workout. Start out doing the plyometrics so that you are fresh and energetic when you do them. Select between three and five of these exercises and perform between 8 and 10 reps per set. Do 2 sets with a 30 second rest between each.

When you are working on your lower-body, bounds, rim jumps, box jumps, jump squats and cone hops are good. If you want to build your upper body's power, you can try using a medicine ball or do plyo pushups.

Rest for two minutes and then get started on the weight training. Keep the exercises to four at most per workout. You could, for example, work the upper body by doing pull-ups, military presses, rows or bench presses.

If it's the lower body you want to work on, step-ups, deadlifts, lunges, and squats should do the trick.

Now, these are just a few of the best-known techniques to develop muscle strength, power, and endurance. You can design your own workout routine by mixing these and continuing to shock your muscles to new levels. Good luck!

Training for Endurance

You can improve your endurance and cardiovascular health through weight training, using a mixture of the techniques that we have gone

The workout samples we gave you in the prior chapter are ready to go. All you need to do is to tailor it for you own goals by changing the number of reps, sets, and intensity. You'll be able to do that now with the information you have learned.

Here's a quick recap:

If you want to build muscle endurance, you have to work on contracting those groups of muscles that you want to develop repeatedly. Circuit training is a good fit here and can use your own body weight to assist.

So, you can, for example, try adding squat thrusts, press-ups, and sit-ups. Work on the muscle areas you want to improve by tailoring your workout – using lunges for lower-body and chest passes for upper-body, for instance.

Circuit training also improves cardiovascular endurance. You can further improve this by including supersets or reducing the time spent resting. Those training for endurance will often use lighter loads in the weight department but a lot more reps.

This is not very effective when it comes to performance, though. It is better to train with heavier weights and reduce the number of reps to improve muscle efficiency.

Training for Strength

Again, you can modify the workouts we provided in the prior chapter to suit your goals in this department.

If you are serious about building strength, you need to use barbells rather than dumbbells or even cable machines. That way you can load a lot more weight. The real way to improve strength is to lift weights. Once you have completed your strength training, then you can start using dumbbells to improve your build.

The shoulder press, bench press, deadlift, and squat are called "The Big Four" for a good reason. They are the very best strength-building exercises. Rowing and chin-ups are also great, but they should not be focused on when exercising. Use them like you would a little seasoning – to improve the flavor, not take it over completely.

If you want to build strength, you need to work on your base and lift heavier weights. You would do, at most, 6 reps per set and limit the number of sets to 4 or 5. You would need to work at, at least 85% of your 1RM doing exercises that engaged multiple joints at once. (Like a bench press or squat.) This is done for 4 weeks in order to make it possible to move on to power training.

There are personal trainers who believe in using a defined speed when doing repetitions, such as three seconds when you are pushing up and one when you are lowering the weight. If you are a beginner, don't bother with that.

Start by getting into the rhythm and making sure that the rep count is accurate. The focus should be on controlled movements and pausing for a second when you are at the top of the lift.

Stick to a rhythm that works well for you or you risk reducing the efficacy of the exercise. Tempo is not as important here as using controlled movements and increasing weight consistently.

You should have no more than 3 to 4 lifts in any particular workout. Shorter workouts make it possible to take full advantage of the hormonal surges that occur. If you try to add in too much per session, there is an above-excellent chance that a few of the exercises will be done half-heartedly.

You really only need one major lift in a workout – that is, one of the Big Four supplemented by a couple of assistance lifts, like chin-ups.

After that, you can work on muscle strengthening and then some exercises designed to target your core or any area that you would like more definition in. Doing more than this is counter-productive and unnecessary.

Change up your rep ranges within your workouts until you find the ideal balance of strength and size gains. Sets of five seem to work well for most people. The big four moves tend to tire you out at about five, so your form might not be consistent after that.

Most people hit the wall and stop progressing because they are using weights that are more heavy than necessary for too long a period. Forget about the guy next to you who is bench pressing more than you are.

Stick to the plan, and you'll soon outstrip him. That means using weights that are around 10% lighter than your maximum weight for the rep range. You can increase it next time, as long as you to stick to increases of, at most, 10 pounds. Keep your form and the same lift schedule, and you will see consistent progress.

The golden rule, as always – what you do to one side, you must do to the other. Keep to that, and you can stay clear of muscle imbalances and injury. Say you decide to do squats to work your quads, do deadlifts to work the hamstrings as well.

When working your chest, work your back as well. Balance work does not have to be executed at the same time as your other exercises, but do make sure it is done within that week.

Following a ratio of two pulling movements to every pushing movement is a good general rule. If you decide to focus on bench-pressing on Monday, for example, make Tuesdays for chin-ups and keep Thursday for lateral raises. This is a practical example of the push-pull formula.

Training for Power

Being able to carry out forceful and quick muscle contractions is what will make it possible to keep good form and reduce injury risk.

Every time you take a step when running, you are absorbing around almost three times what your total bodyweight is in force. You then need to push yourself off to make the next stride possible.

If you haven't prepared properly for this, you are bound to injure yourself. Plyometrics and heavy lifting can aid in reducing reaction time on the ground and so also improve your performance and reduce exercise risk.

To develop power, you need high sets, with low reps and heavy weight. You could try 4 to 5 sets, each with 3 reps; 5 to 6 sets, each with 1 or 2 reps; or as much as 7 to 8 sets each with only one rep.

Increasing your strength and power and lifting more weight is something anyone can do, provided you lift sensibly and are prepared to work hard.

1. Lift heavier. The best way of increasing your strength and power on a lift is to lift heavier weights.
2. Lift less.
3. Lift correctly.
4. Add variety.

Powerlifting and weightlifting training are great but very specific ways to train for power. Performing a deadlift involves a strong base of strength, whereas a movement like the snatch requires explosive power.

If you are just starting out, or if you are a bit more practiced but not too far advanced, you can see immediate gains if you try the periodization technique.

This simply means setting goals within your training schedule and putting a date to them. You can incorporate strength training, body building, etc.

If you are pretty far advance, however, you need to keep your focus on building power. If you want more advice on periodization methods, just conduct a little research – there are many methods out there. Choose the one that suits you the best.

A fatal error that those looking to increase their power make is to add to great an amount of volume and then not resting enough.

If you are doing just 1 or 2 reps at a time and have a good rest of between 3 and 4 minutes between each set, you are not going to feel as tired or as sore.

This may give you the impression that the workout wasn't effective. This is a false impression. If you try and push further too fast, you will delay your progress.

Power lifting requires a controlled level of volume and a good rest between sets so that you can give each rep 100% effort.

Now it's time for you to put together your workout program based on the samples I provided in the previous chapter and modify to your needs.

I hope you have learned something from this book so far and would greatly appreciate it if you could leave an honest review on Amazon.com.

Chapter 7

The Moves

This chapter provides a guide to the exercises listed in this book, sorted by the major body part that the exercise focuses on. There are hundreds of exercises available, but I only listed the best ones you need as the foundation of your fitness program. The rest are mostly just variations of these.

Chest Exercises

Barbell Bench Press

This is a compound press that works out the full body. Your triceps, shoulders, and chest get the most work. This is the best exercise if you want to both improve the muscle mass and strength in your upper-body. This involves lifting the heaviest set of weights and will be something that you will continue with throughout your journey.

1. Sit down on the end of the bench. It should be completely flat. Once in position, lower your back until you are fully prone with your back on the bench.

2. Squeeze together the shoulder blades and the lift your chest. Tighten the muscles in your upper-back. Get a firm grip on the bar and place your little finger on the inside of the ring marks.

3. Get your feet ready by making sure they are shoulder-width apart and flat on the floor. Lift the bar with your arms straight.

4. With a controlled, slow movement, bring it down towards your chest. In a controlled, slow movement, straighten your arms again until the elbows lock. That's one rep.

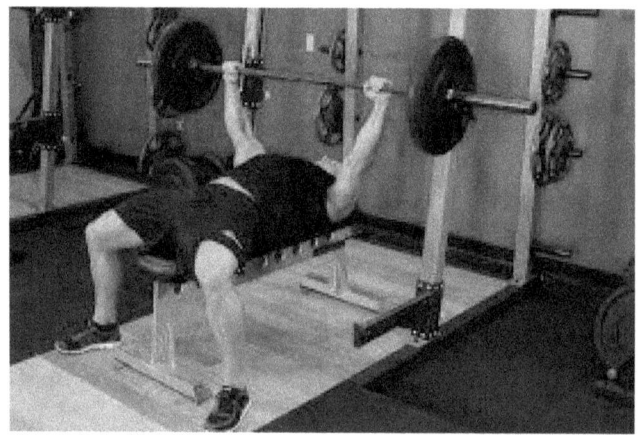

Remember:

-*Only do one or two sets.*

-*Choose between 8 and 15 reps - vary the pattern on a regularly.*

-*This should be done only once every week.*

-*Keep your grip tight and about shoulder-width apart.*

-*The lowest point for the bar is when it touches your chest.*

Incline Dumbbell Press

This works on strengthening your upper-body. Your triceps, should and chest will get a workout. The bench is inclined here to more effectively target your shoulders and upper chest.

Free weights are more suitable because they allow more range of motion and minimize differences in the strengths of the arms.

1. Incline the bench to 30 or 45 degrees. Settle in, making sure that your back is fully supported. Hold your arms with the free weights in them directly up so that the elbows lock.

2. Pull together the shoulder blades and stick your chest out a little. Bring the free weights down in a slow, controlled movement until they are level with your chest.

3. Hold for a second and then move back to your starting position slowly.

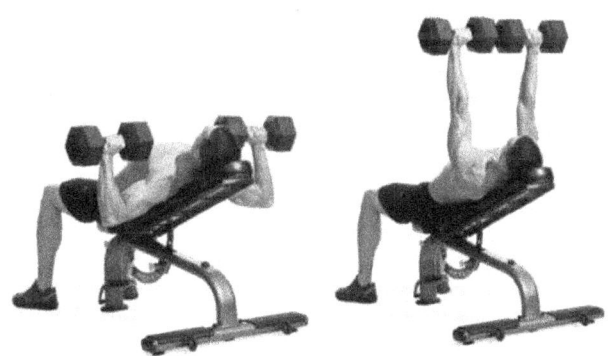

Remember:

-Your elbows must be tucked in close to the body when possible.

-Be wary of overextending your neck. Keep the movement in the shoulders, not the neck.

Incline Chest Fly

A dumbbell fly is an exercise for your upper body. To allow your elbows to move behind your torso, you should do the exercise on a bench.

A dumbbell fly will primarily work muscles in your chest and shoulders; however, it will have some strengthening effect on other muscles in your back and arms as well.

You can do either incline or flat bench chest fly. The incline fly targets the upper chest more. You can also vary this exercise by using cables or barbell instead of dumbbells.

1. Set your incline bend to 30 degrees maximum. Hold a dumbbell in each of your hands. Lay down on the bench. Straighten your arms upwards, bending the elbows slightly – and bring your palms together.

2. Change the position of your hands so that the knuckles face each other, and your pinkies are next to each other. Inhale and bring your arms down in a slow, controlled movement. At the same time, change the position of your hands so that the palms face one another again.

3. Exhale and start raising your arms again, once again changing the orientation of your hands. Repeat as required.

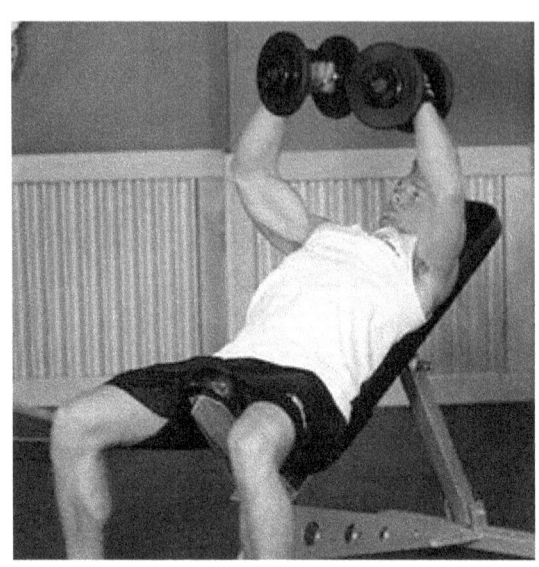

Remember:

-*The pinky fingers should be next to each other. This will be your starting position.*

-*At the end of the movement, the arms will be by your side with the palms facing the ceiling.*

-*Keep in mind that the movement will only happen at the shoulder joint and the wrist. There is no motion that happens at the elbow joint.*

Machine Chest Press

This is different to bench pressing in that you are not lying down to do it. This is great for those with shoulder injuries because you can change the handles' angles. This allows you to work with minimal risk of further inflaming your shoulder.

1. Sit with your back completely supported by the backrest and your feet flush with the floor or footrest. Grip the handles and pull forward until you have straightened your arms completely.

2. Hold for a second or so and then start pulling your arms back in a controlled motion to get you back to the starting point.

3. Do 4 sets with about 8 to 12 reps in each and rest for a minute when each set is done.

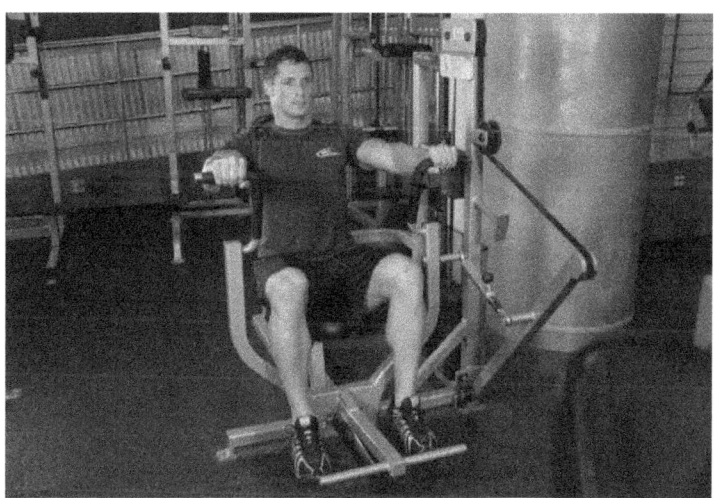

Back Exercises

Chin-up (also called pull-up)

The chin-up helps to strengthen your body. It works the muscles of the back and the biceps.

1. Grip the bar keeping your hands shoulder-width apart and your palms facing down. Bend your knees a little, so you are hanging for a little, arms completely straight.

2. Now you can start the exercise. Lift your body by pulling up, keeping your elbows close to the body. Raise yourself until your chin is above the bar – don't cheat!

3. Lower yourself down again, keeping your feet off the floor, until your arms have straightened out again. Inhale and repeat.

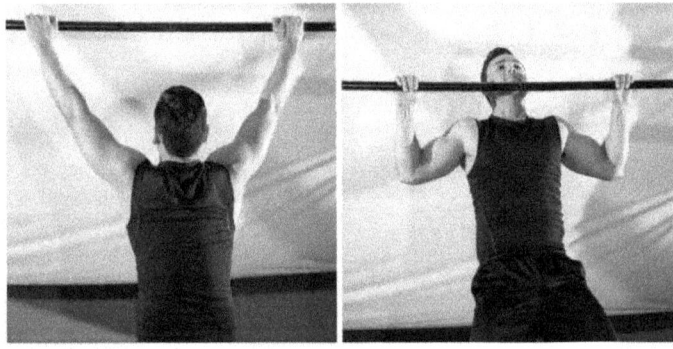

Remember:

-Pull-ups look a lot easier than they are. If you cannot do a full pull-up, start doing negatives. Stand on something that gives

you enough height to get your chin to the right height and then lower yourself, making sure that your feet are hanging free.

-When you want to go back up again, put your feet on the bench again and start again.

-Alternatively, use a resistance band to give your legs more support or ask someone to assist by holding onto your legs.

Seated Cable Row

This exercise helps to isolate the upper and middle back and improve them. It is also a great way to improve balance in your shoulder muscles and improves posture.

1. Sit down and place your feet on the attached platform. Grip the handle with palms facing together.

2. Lean back, so that your arms are straight, being sure that your feet are supporting you. Bring the handle towards you by bending your elbows.

3. When it is as close to you as possible, squeeze together your shoulder blades and hold for a second or two. Then return to the position you started in.

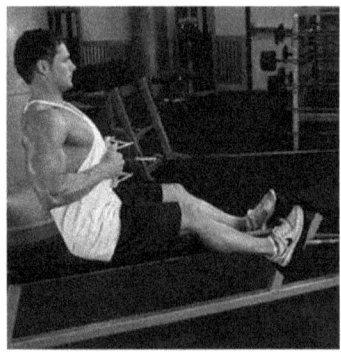

Remember:

-You must lean backwards, not forwards.

-Keep your back upright and do not move your torso when pulling.

Single Arm Dumbbell Row

This exercise is a variation of the row exercises that work the lower back muscles with some benefit to the biceps and forearms. It is especially useful if you are dealing with a back injury.

1. Stand to the right of your weight bench. Using your right hand, grip a dumbbell with your palm facing your body.

2. Place your left knee and your left hand on top of the bench for support. Extend your right arm and let it hang a little to the front.

3. Pull your abdominals in and bend forward from the hips so that your back is naturally arched and roughly parallel to the floor, and your right knee is slightly bent.

4. Tuck in your chest until your neck lines up with your spinal column. Raise your right arm until you have your elbow facing the ceiling, your upper arm is parallel to the floor, and your hand comes to the outside of the ribcage. Lower in a slow, controlled movement.

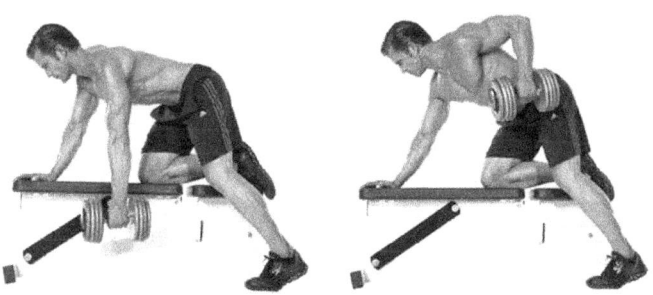

Remember:

-Focus on using your back muscles to pull rather than just using your arms.

-Keep your core tight for added support.

-Don't allow your back to start sagging towards the floor and don't hunch your shoulders.

-Pull your shoulders back and down to set the shoulder blades.

Deadlift

Deadlifting will support your aesthetic goals, help you build better posture, correct various strength imbalances, help you build total strength. It is one of the most effective exercises for developing the pure strength that's a precursor to bodily size and athleticism.

1. Get your stance right by placing the middle of your feet directly underneath the bar, with feet hip-width apart. Don't let it touch your shins for now. Place your feet facing out at around a 15-degree angle.

2. Grip the bar. Keeping your legs straight and place your hands shoulder-width apart. You may now bend the knees. Continue until your shins are touching the bar and without moving it forward at all. If it rolls forward, you must start over.

3. Start raising your chest. This will help to make your back muscles stronger. Other than that, make no changes in position.

4. Lift. Inhale deeply and hold it while you are lifting the weight. The bar should still be in contact with your legs. Be careful bit to throw yourself backwards or to shrug. Lock the knees and the hips.

5. Unlock your knees and then hips and start to lower the bar to the floor. Once it moves over your knees, you can start bending them properly. The bar should end up in the same position it started in.

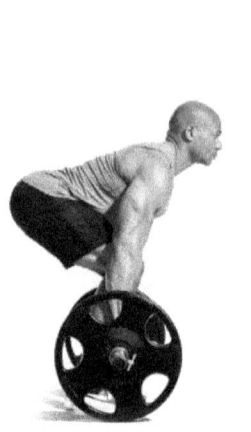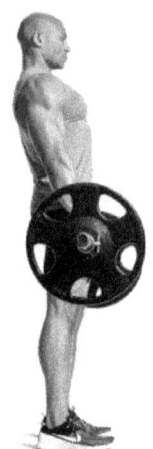

Remember:

-Try to use your legs to help push.

-A one second rest is all you need between each rep. Rest in the starting position, gripping the bar. Inhale deeply and repeat the exercise.

-Do not allow the weight to bounce when it hits the floor, or you will start damaging your form.

Shoulder Exercises

Clean and Press

This is an Olympic lift and helps to strengthen the whole body. Your shoulders are the main focus of this workout, but your calves, hamstrings, quadriceps, glutes, abdominals, lower and middle back and traps also get worked out. Your whole body is worked out, and you can use this both for muscle building and increasing strength.

1. Stand with your feet shoulder-width. Make sure that your shins are around two inches from the barbell. Grip the barbell while pushing your hips back. Your palms should be facing you, and your hands should also be shoulder-width apart. Your arms must be completely straight, and your butt should be tucked in.

2. Hold your core in and then lift, using your heels to give the main support. Make sure that your chest is kept tall. When the bar is just above knee-height, you should extend the hips, knees, and ankles explosively. Shrug the shoulders and keep the bar as near to your body as you can.

3. Bend your knees and bring the bar up to shoulder height. You will have to change the positions of your hands so that the palms face away from you and that means releasing the bar for a split second.

4. When you have changed position, straighten the knees and extend the bar over your head until your arms are completely straight again.

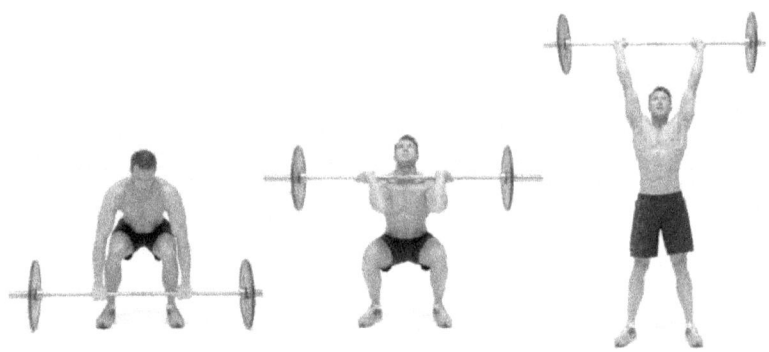

Remember:

-Your hamstrings glutes and hips should be used to pull the bar up to the height of your chest.

-You must let your heels support your weight at all times.

-You must keep your upper back straight and not rounded as you lift.

Push Press

This exercise is a compound one that is also dynamic. It helps to increase the power and strength of both halves of the body. It focuses on the core, hips, and shoulders.

It is similar in natural to a military press, but the "push" comes from the legs. You then lower the weight a bit at a time to chest-level. Alternatively, you can incorporate just after you have done a squat, by keeping it behind your neck.

1. Grip the barbell with hands just a little closer together than shoulder-width apart. Hoist it to a position that is a little over shoulder-height, keeping your elbows tucked close to your body for support. Bend at the knees, so you are half squatting.

2. Start pushing the legs so that you explosively straighten them, while lifting the barbell up and over your head. Your arms should be fully extended. Hold for a second and then bring it back down to the shoulders.

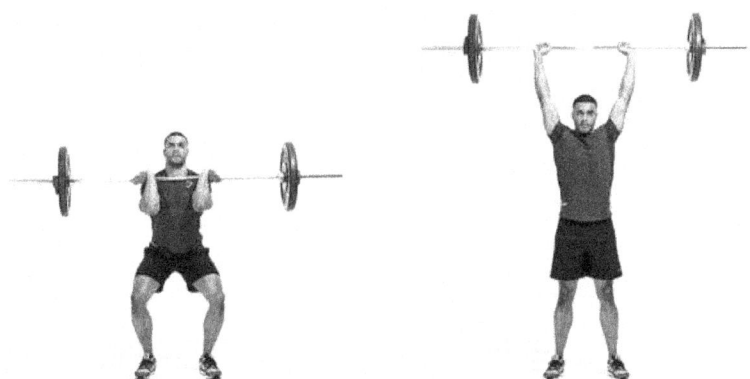

Remember:

-Doing this explosively using the legs and hips to get the movement going will give the best results.

-Take care that you don't hyperextend your back.

-Lock your elbows at the highest point for maximum support.

Snatch

The snatch is one of two lifts in the sport of weightlifting. The objective of the snatch is to lift the barbell from the ground to overhead in one continuous motion. This is a power exercise that builds overall explosiveness.

1. Line up your feet under the bar, hip-width apart. Grip the bar keeping hands at least 30 inches apart. This will depend on how tall you are and how flexible you are. — 30-plus inches, depending on your height and shoulder flexibility. Squat down, keeping your back and arms straight and be sure to squat low enough that your knees are lower than your hips.

2. Start lifting using your back, glutes, and legs. Make sure that your shins are close to the bar but not in contact with it. Once you have lifted it just above knee-height, use every ounce of power to accelerate the lift. Keep the weight on your toes.

3. When it is above your head, shrug your shoulders and move so that you are in front of the bar and doing a complete squat. Shift your wrists and push up until your arms are completely extended, and the elbows lock. You may need to widen your stance a little.

4. Give yourself a second to ensure that the barbell is completely balanced and stand up, ensuring that the bar lines up with your hips and ankles. In a controlled movement, put the barbell down.

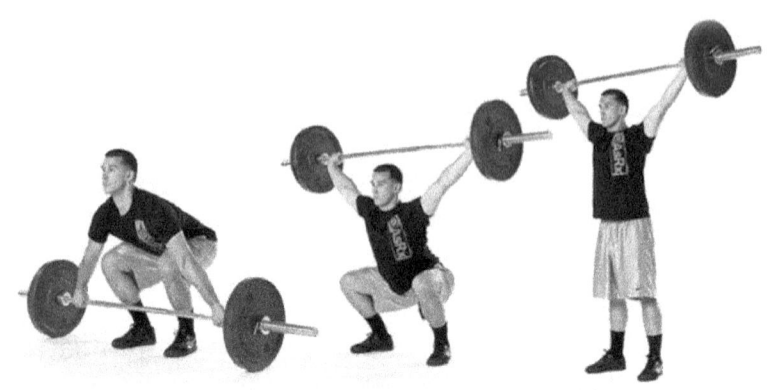

Side Lateral Raise

The side lateral raise is an isolation exercise that strengthens the entire shoulder with an emphasis on the sides of the deltoid muscles. You can vary the angle of bend of your body to make the exercise stricter. The heavier the weights, the more you will have to lean forward.

1. Grip the dumbbells so that they are in front of your thighs and bend your elbows slightly. Bend a little and keep knees and hips a little bent.

2. Lift your arms until they are fully extended to the side, and the elbows are at the same levels as your shoulder. Without locking your elbows.

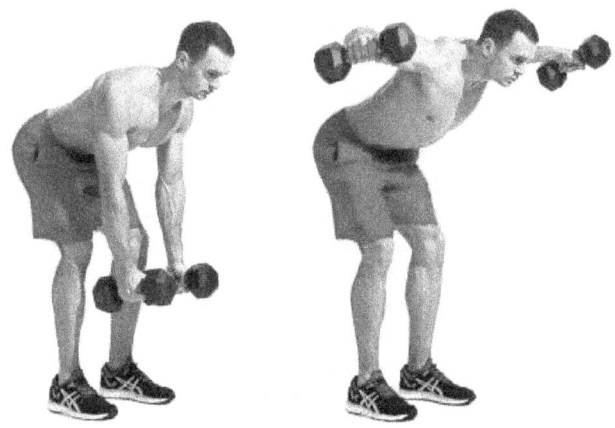

Remember:

-Your elbows should be slightly bent at all times.

-It's important that your elbows match shoulder-height to target the lateral deltoids. Your dumbbell should always be a little lower than the shoulders.

-Bending your torso helps to target the lateral deltoids better.

Arnold Dumbbell Press

This is an alternative to the normal shoulder press. It is named for Arnold Schwarzenegger because he used it in building his shoulder muscles.

During the press section of your lift, you will have to use rotational movement and this, in turn, make the shoulder more stable. You will work the shoulder muscles on the inside at the lowest point of your lift.

1. Grip your dumbbells. Raise them till they are level with your shoulder, keeping your elbows bent and your palms facing towards you.

2. Hold your dumbbells as tight as you can manage and then raise them over your head. Rotate them as you do so so that your palms face away from you when your arms are fully extended.

3. Hold for a second, and then start to lower the weight. As you do so, rotate your hands again so that they are facing you again.

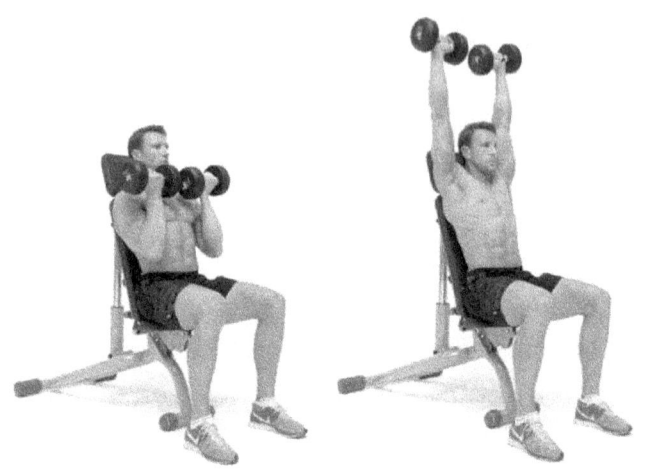

Remember:

-Slow, controlled movements are best.

-Make sure that you fully rotate the weight.

Leg Exercises

Barbell Squat

The barbell squats are your bread and butter to stronger and bigger legs, whatever level you are. Squats are one of the best exercises to work your core and lower body.

If you schedule them in on a regular basis, they will help to create definition in the buttocks and thighs. They can be done anywhere because your body acts as the "weight." Digestion, circulation, and posture can all be improved with squats. They are low impact and easy to do.

1. Start by gripping the bar well and dip under it to transfer the weight to behind your ears. Keep your feet under it. Lift the bar off the rack by standing up. Lock your knees and hips.

2. Take a deep breath and squat. Your knees should be pushed out as your hips are moving back. Your lower back should be kept in neutral.

3. Deepen the squat until your thighs are in a parallel position compared to the floor. Stand up again and breath.

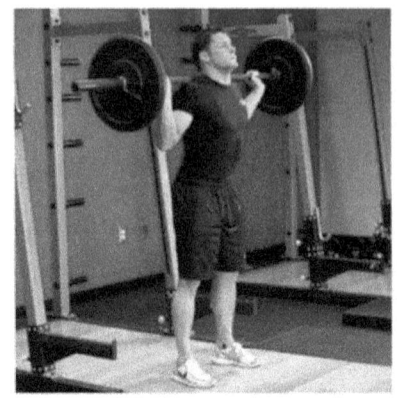 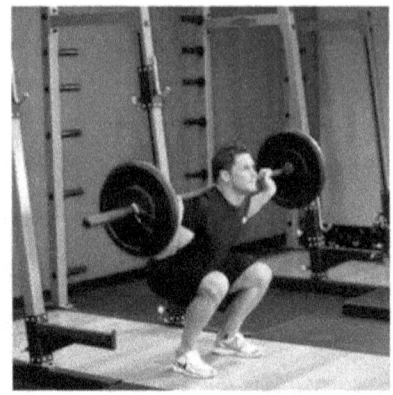

Remember:

-If you want to up the intensity, you can go lower with the squat.

-You should explode on your way back up.

-Don't ever let your knees go further than your toes.

Half-Squat

The half squat is an exercise for those with intermediate level of physical fitness and exercise experience. It can also be used by non-beginners to force the body to handle much heavier weights than the regular squats and thus stimulate the nervous system to release growth hormones. It's a fitness hack.

1. Get in position with your feet should-width apart and yourself under the bar. The bar should not rest on the nape of your neck, but rather on your shoulders.

2. Hold the bar using a wider grip. Bend your knees and straighten up your back. Push your body up so that you can lift the weight, keeping your back straight.

3. Step back a little and get the weight balanced. Lower yourself down, keeping your back straight and not leaning forward.

4. Do a half-squat, hold for a second and then push back up again. Do not allow your knees to lock when you are in the full upright position.

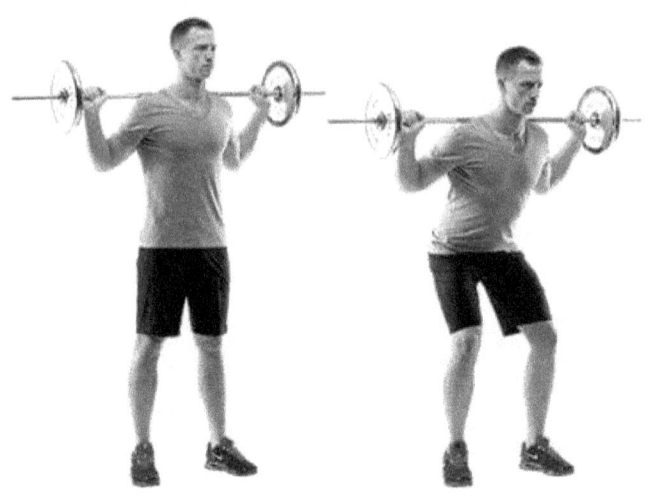

Remember:

-This exercise should only be used as a shock technique.

-It is best to do the regular squat exercise before doing the half squat as this is only a supplemental exercise.

Hamstring Curl

Also called lying leg curls, this exercise is the top exercise for directly working the hamstrings.

1. Maintain a taut torso. Strengthen your core muscles to make this easier.

2. Make sure that you have your legs completely stretched when starting. Get a hold of the handles that are directly in front of you for support. Breathe out and then curl your legs.

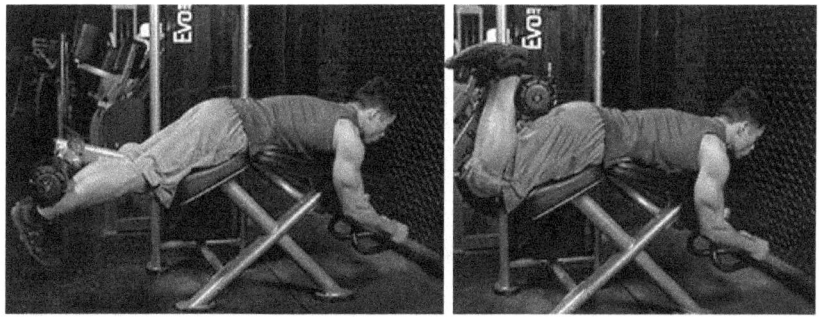

Remember:

-It is better to make use of an angled leg curl machine because this improves the stretch to the hamstrings.

Single Leg Press

Doing leg presses using only one leg means that you activate more muscle and get better benefits in terms of the range of motion. It looks a lot like a standard leg press, but it doesn't feel like one.

1. Get into position on the machine and make sure that you have one foot on the floor and the other on the bar.

2. Lower the bar until your knee is at right angles to the floor. Using the heel of your foot, push back to the starting position.

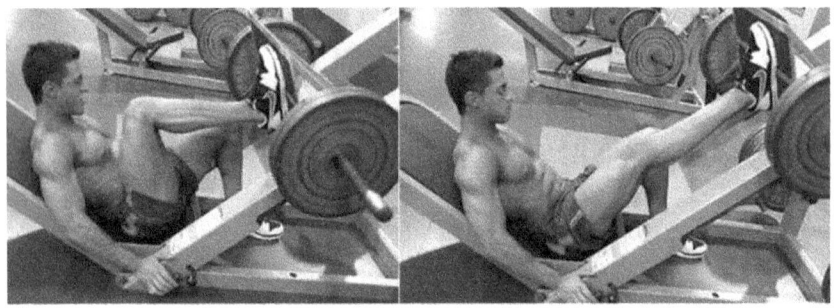

Leg Extension

The leg extension targets the quadriceps muscle in the legs. The exercise is done using a machine called the Leg Extension Machine.

1. Get into position on the machine. Your legs will go underneath the pad, and your toes will point forwards. Hold the bars on the side for more stability.

2. Your start position is when the upper and lower legs are at right angles to each other. This is very important, or you risk injuring your knee.

3. Bring your lower legs up so that they are fully extended. Hold for a second. Lower them in a slow, controlled motion.

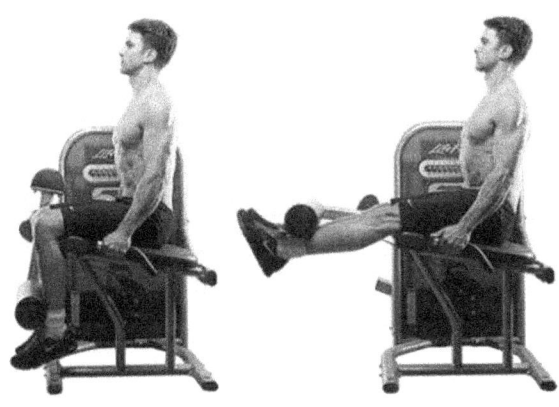

Dumbbell Lunge

The targeted muscles include the glutes in your hips and butt along with the hamstrings and quadriceps in your thighs. The calf muscles in your lower legs, the abdominal muscles, and the back muscles act as stabilizers during this exercise.

1. Select your dumbbells and stand straight up, bending your knees a little. Keep your arms with the dumbbells in them next to your side. This is the start position.

2. Stride forward with one leg, keeping balanced and then squat into the lunge.

3. Make sure that your core is stable and keep the movement limited to the legs. Keep the knee above the toes. Push back up to the start and repeat on the other side.

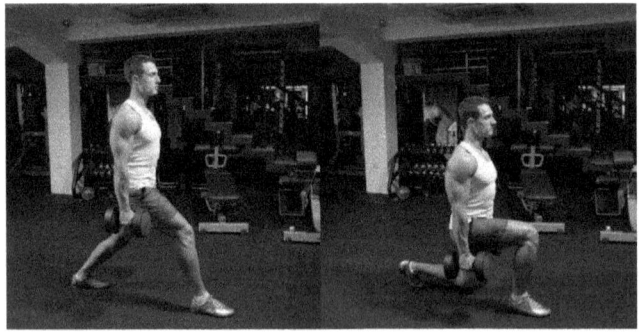

Remember:

-*Your knees should never go out in front of the toes, or you will stress the joints.*

-If you are not good at balancing, this is not a good exercise for you.

-Never round your back.

Bicep Exercises

Barbell Curls

This is an isolation move that only works one joint. Your biceps are targeted, but you will find that some of the smaller muscles in your arm are also worked out.

1. Keep your back up straight and grip your barbell with hands shoulder-width apart. Your palms should face you, and you keep your elbows as close to your side as possible.

2. Bend the elbows and lift the weight. This is the start position. Lower the weight while inhaling. Only the forearms need to move here.

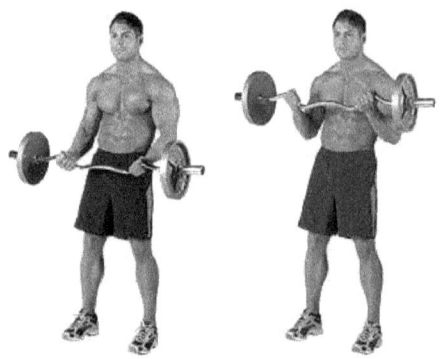

Remember:

-You can use EZ curls to help with grip and the position of your wrist.

-Alternatively, use a cable machine for this.

Single Arm Bench Bicep Curls

You can also call this the one-arm dumbbell preacher curl.

1. Grip your dumbbell using your right arm. Position your upper arm on the machine or an incline bench. It must be a shoulder length away from you. This is the start.

2. Inhale and start to drop the dumbbell slowly until your arm is completely extended and you feel the stretch in your biceps.

3. Exhale and start to raise the dumbbell until the biceps have contracted completely and the weight is level with your shoulder. Tightly squeeze the biceps before returning to the start position. Repeat with the other arm.

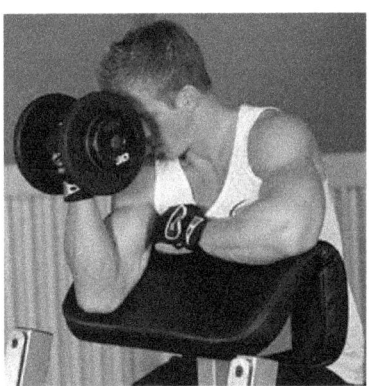

Remember:

-This can be done on a low pulley machine instead. You'll just need to change the bench's position.

-Add in extra reps using your other hand as support. Be sure that your movement is completely controlled though.

Dumbbell Alternate Bicep Curl with Twist

1. Keeping your back straight, grip dumbbells in both hands at the length of your arms. Tuck your elbows close to the side. Your palms should face towards your thighs.

2. Keeping your upper arm still, bend the elbow of one arm and raise the weight. At the same time, rotate your hand so that it is facing forward.

3. Keep it there for a couple of seconds and tighten the biceps more. Reverse your movements so that you are back to the start. Repeat on the other side.

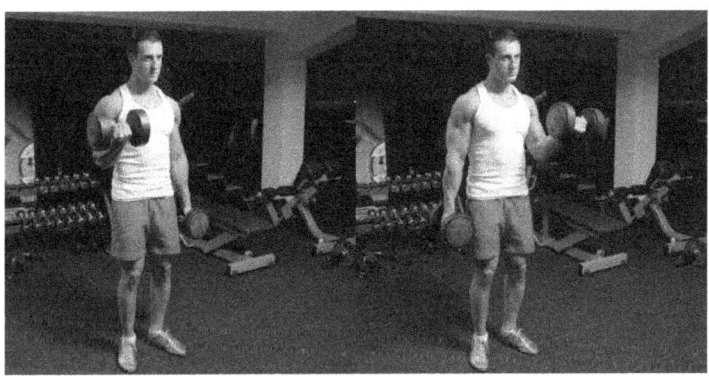

Remember:

-You can change this up a lot of ways – you could sit and use back support, or sit on a plain bench. You could save time by doing it on both sides at once. Alternatively, do all the curls on one side and then do the other side.

-You can also change the position of your palms

Overhead Cable Curls

This is also known as a High Cable Curl, and it works your biceps through the use of a cable.

The cable is usually set level with your shoulder, sometimes higher, and this isolates your biceps and allows for a better contraction.

1. Start off by making sure that you have weights on that are comfortable for you. The weights on either side should match. Change the pulley's height so that it is level with or higher than your shoulder.

2. Position yourself in the center and grip the handles with your palms facing up at the ceiling and your feet shoulder-width apart. Your arms ought to be parallel to the ceiling and completely extended. Make sure that both sides are about equal. This is where you start.

3. Exhale and, while doing so, squeeze your biceps and curl until your bicep is fully contracted.

4. Inhale and return to the start position. This is a completely stationary exercise – your arms should be doing the heavy lifting.

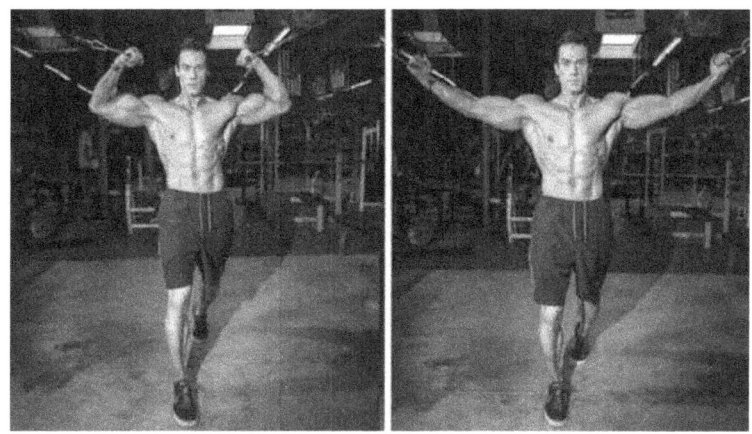

Remember:

-While curling the muscle, make sure you feel the biceps contracting strongly. This is what is going to benefit you the most.

Triceps Exercises

Cable Triceps Pushdown

1. This is done using a high pulley system. Grip the bar with your palms facing the floor and hands shoulder-width apart.

2. Stand up straight, leaning forward a little and pull down so that your upper arms are tucked in next to your body. Your elbows should be bent, and your forearms should face forwards. You should look a little like a dog begging for a treat. This is the start.

3. Now exhale and lower the bar until you touch your thighs and your arms are completely extended and almost at a right angle to the floor. Move only your forearms here. Hold for about a second, inhale and return to the start position.

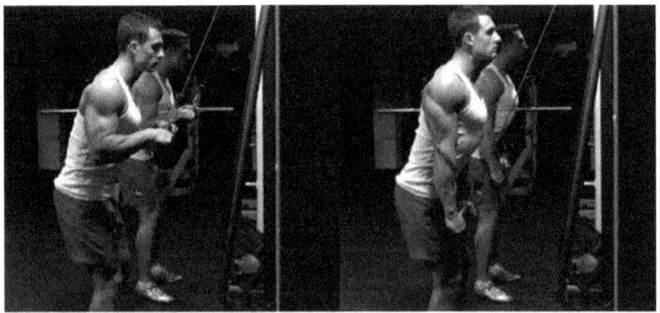

Remember:

-You can vary this exercise in many different ways. Use a machine that lets you swap out the handles. Use the E-Z bar or

a V-angled bar so that your thumb stays higher up than your pinkie. This helps to stretch the muscle further. Alternatively, just use a rope or reverse grip to change things up.

-There are many variations to this movement. For instance, you can use an E-Z bar attachment as well as a V-angled bar that allows the thumb to be higher than the small finger. Also, you can attach a rope to the pulley as well as using a reverse grip on the bar exercises.

Incline EZ Bar Lying Triceps Extension

1. Grip your barbell with your palms facing down and at slightly less than shoulder-width apart. Set the incline bench at 45 to 75 degrees and lay down on it.

2. The barbell should be brought overhead. Keep your elbows in and extend your arms throughout. Your arms should line up with your torso and be above your head. This is the start position.

3. Inhale and start lowering the barbell using a semicircular movement. You will be moving it away from you until your biceps and forearms meet. Again, making sure that your forearms do all the moving.

4. Exhale and go back to the start. Contract your triceps muscle and hold for about a second.

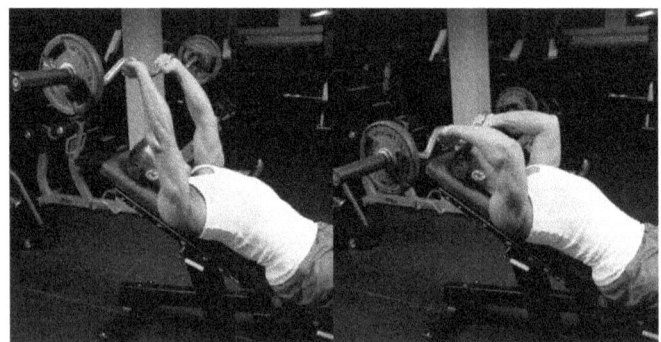

Remember:

-You can use an E-Z bar here, two dumbbells, or do it sitting or standing to vary the exercise.

Dumbbell One-Arm Triceps Extension

1. Grip your dumbbell and get into position. You can use a utility bench if it supports your back or use a military press bench instead. Alternatively, you could stand up straight.

2. Bring the dumbbell first to shoulder height and then extend it up fully, keeping it close to your head.

3. You can use the other hand to support your upper arm, keep it at your side or grab a support with it. Turn your wrist so your palm faces forwards and little finger faces upwards. This is the start position.

4. Lower your dumbbell slowly past your shoulder blades behind you. Breathe in when doing this and pause for a second when you feel a good stretch in the triceps. Exhale and slowly reverse your movements.

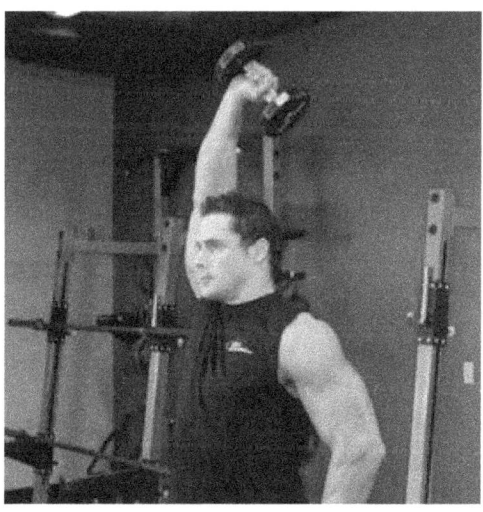

Remember:

-I sound like a stuck record, but only your forearm should move.

-This can also be done with a rope.

Calf Exercises

Standing Calf Raise

These exercise the tibialis, gastrocnemius, soleus and posterior muscles in your lower leg. An ankle extension is the basic movement at play here.

1. Climb onto a step and stand at the very edge of it. The only parts of the foot that should touch it are the balls of the feet and toes. You can also use a platform for step-aerobics but will have to use a couple of risers to raise it.

2. Stand up straight and make sure that your core is fully engaged. Keep the abdominal muscles tight. Let your heels hang over the edge.

3. If necessary, stand near the wall or something you can grab onto if balance becomes a problem for you. Lift your heels up so that you end up standing on tiptoes on the edge of the platform or step.

4. Hold for about a second or two and then drop your heels in a slow, controlled motion until you can feel your calves stretching out nicely. If need be, stabilize yourself by hanging on a wall or some other stationary object.

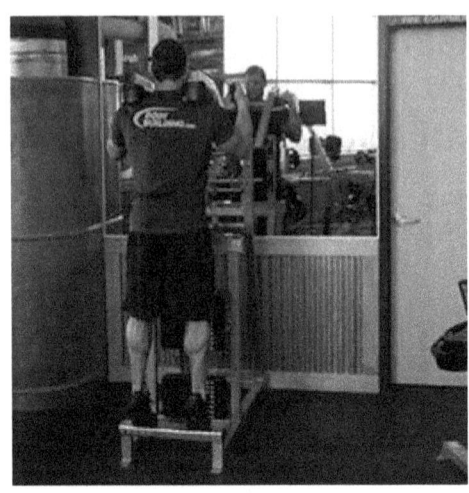

Remember:

-Make the difference as noticeable as you can. Go as high as you can go and then drop down as low as you can. The more you can do, the better.

-Make sure that you do push off evenly. All the toes should be engaged for this, or you risk injuring one or two of them.

Seated Calf Raise

1. Get into position and put your toes in the correct place on the lower platform. (Look for something that looks like pedals on a bike but that are fixed in place.) Choose the position of the toe that suits you best.

2. Your thighs will have to be placed underneath the pad – you may have to adjust the lever to keep it in place. Push your heels up and release any safety bars. This will make the lever rise a bit, and this is your start position.

3. Lower the heels again until you can feel the stretch in your calves. Breath in while stretching the calves and out while contracting them. Hold for about a second or so and then return to the start position.

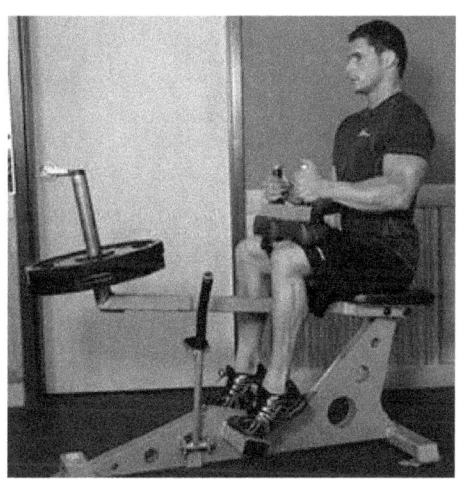

Abdominal Exercises

Crunch

1. Lay on the floor with your hands placed on your stomach, palms facing downwards. Bend your knees and lift your feet off the floor slightly. Alternatively, lift them straight up into the air.

2. Raise your hips off the ground using only your abdominal muscles. Contract the abdominal muscles while doing so and hold for a couple of seconds. Let go and return to the starting position slowly.

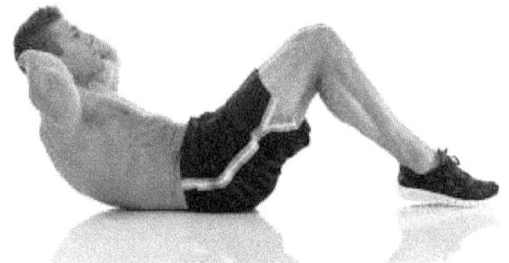

Reverse Crunch

1. Lay on the floor and place your palms on the ground. Move your knees so that they are at a ninety-degree angle to your hips with your feet raised a little off the ground. This is the start position.

2. Using your abdominals, raise the hips from the floor. Hold for a second or two and then lower them again. You should not, however, let your feet touch the floor – they should hover just above it.

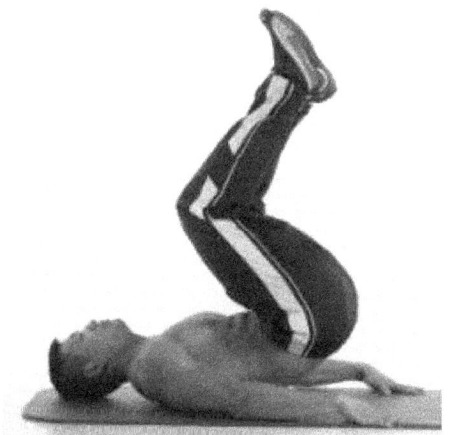

Leg Raise

1. Lay on a bend with your legs stretched out in front of you. Your hand position is up to you, you can either hold your hands behind your back, palms facing the bench, or you can hold the bench's sides for extra support. This is your start position.

2. Being sure to keep the legs as straight as you can, bend the knees a little a little and lift up your legs so that they form a ninety-degree angle to your abdomen, exhaling all the way.

3. Hold it for about a second and then inhale and reverse your movements until you are back at the start position.

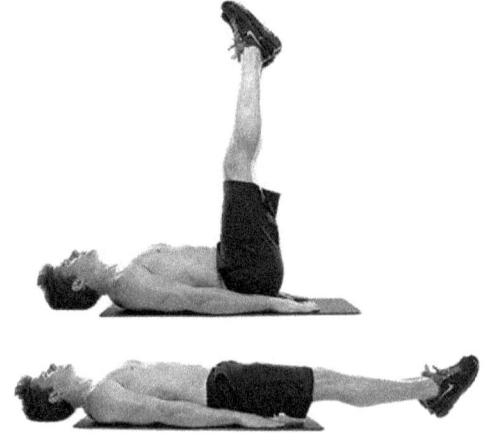

Remember:

-You don't need a bench for this; you can just lay on the floor instead.

-To up the intensity when this becomes a little tame, grip a dumbbell with your feet and raise it when you raise your legs.

-Another way of upping the intensity is to do this exercise straight after a chin-up. You can hang on the bar and do it.

Bicycle Crunch

1. Lay down on the floor and stretch out your legs. Keep your arms straight along the side of your body. Take time getting the form right here, or you won't like the results.

2. You can now lock your fingers behind your head or just hold them there if that's more comfortable.

3. Start lifting your legs and bend the knees. Your thighs should be at right angles to the ground, and your calves should be parallel to the ceiling. At this stage, your feet should be kept together.

4. Bring your right knee back a little and twist your upper body up so that the left elbow touches it. While you are doing this, stretch out your right leg, so it is completely parallel to the floor.

5. Do not let the outstretched leg touch the floor and hold for a second. Return to the start position and repeat on the other side.

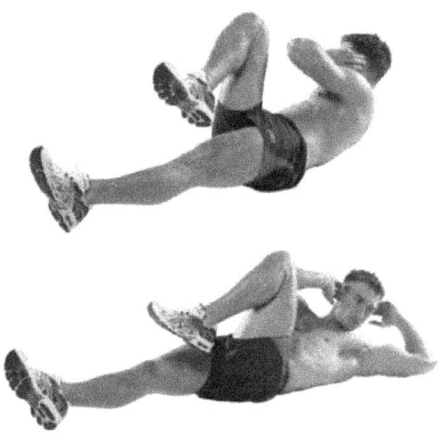

Remember:

-You need to engage your core here, or your neck is going to do a lot of the work. This defeats the whole purpose of the exercise. Use your abs like you are supposed to.

-Never let your feet rest either on your body or the ground during this exercise, keep the muscles controlled and tensed.

-Don't cheat by bringing your elbows closer together when doing the crunch. Keep them in a straight line and in line with your head at all times.

Vertical Leg Raise

1. Hanging Leg Raise – To do this, you need to make sure you're your legs are as straight as possible. You then need to bend at the hip and raise your legs and thighs so that they are parallel to the ceiling. Tighten your core muscles before doing this and keep your legs straight and together.

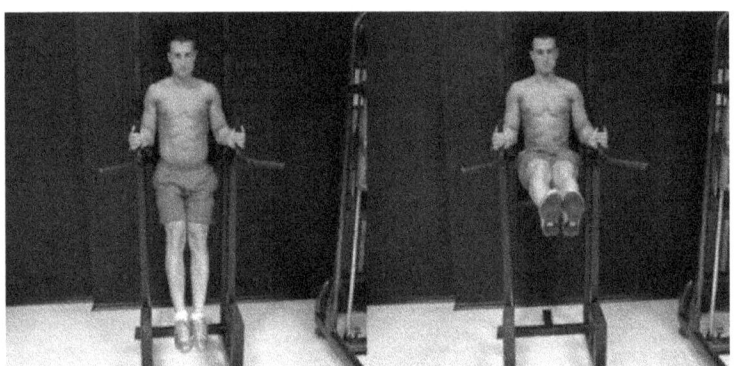

Plank

1. Lie down on the floor as if you are going to do a pushup. Get up onto your elbows, making sure that they are at a ninety-degree angle to the floor. Your forearms are what will support your weight.

2. Rise up onto tiptoes so that your body as straight as you can get it and hold for as long as you can.

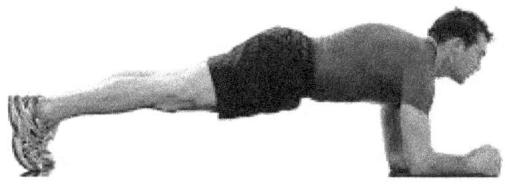

Remember:

-This is a deceptively simple exercise so don't be disheartened if you don't manage to hold it for long.

Decline Reverse Crunch

1. Set up a decline bench and lay down on it. Grip the bench on top and hold your body in this position. It must not slip at all.

2. Your legs should be slightly bent and fully extended, feet just a little above the floor. This is the start position.

3. Exhale and then raise your legs up towards your chest. Roll your pelvis so that you are able to get your hips right off the bench. You are done when your legs are as close to your chest as possible.

4. Hold for a second and then inhale and slowly return to your start position.

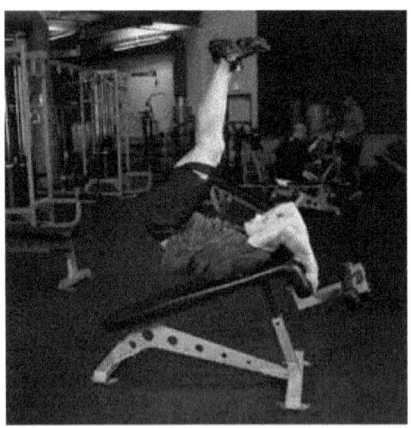

Remember:

-You can also do this using a flat bench.

-To up the intensity, add ankle weights.

Ab Wheel Rollout

1. Kneel down on the floor and pick up your Ab Roller with both hands. Put it directly ahead of you. Move forward until you look like you are doing a kneeling push-up. This is the start position.

2. Inhale deeply and roll forward slowly and feel the stretch in your body. You want to roll forward as far as possible without actually having anything more than your knees and the Ab Roller touching the ground.

3. Pause for about a second or so and then reverse back to the start position in slow, controlled movements. Keep your abdominals engaged throughout the exercise.

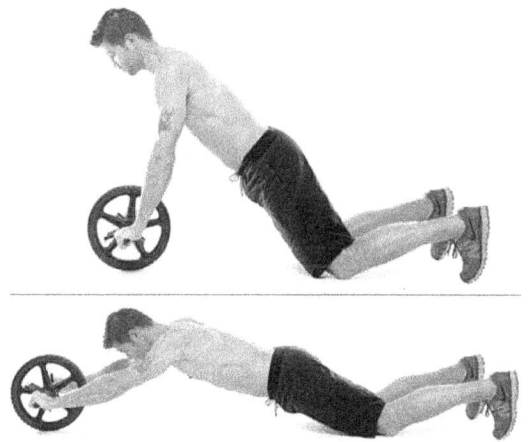

Remember:

-If you have problems with your back, particularly your lower back, skip this one.

-If you have a hernia, skip this one.

-To increase the intensity of the exercise, you can move to the side rather than straight out ahead. This works your obliques more.

Don't forget to share your thoughts on this book by leaving a review on Amazon.com. It takes just a few seconds.

Chapter 8

Nutrition

When you are bodybuilding or weight training, you need to pay as much attention to the food you eat as you do to the training your put in. If you don't get the right nutrients, your body won't be able to repair itself and progress will stall.

The subject of nutrition could fill several books, so I am just going to give you the basics. Once you have an idea, you can research the topic as you please. Here is what you must know to start off with:

1. You will need protein, and you will need lots of it. Research how much you need to maintain your weight and how much you need to add muscle mass.

2. If you are hungry between meals, use a liquid supplement.

3. Don't ever, EVER skip a meal.

4. Make sure that your diet is balanced and that you are getting enough of the other macro-nutrients as well.

5. Drink enough water for your body mass. On a high protein diet, this is even more important.

6. Keep tabs on your fat intake – you cannot go crazy with it, or you won't be able to see the muscles under it.

7. Steer clear of junk food and foods that are processed.

8. Sugar is off the table completely and so are sweets.

Lean proteins are good for you. Choose good quality proteins to assist in building muscles fast.

To roughly work out how much protein, you should eat in a day, multiply your bodyweight in pounds by a total of 0.8. This will tell you how many grams of protein you need to eat in any one day.

To find out what your overall calorie count is, you can check out a calorie calculator online. You plug in your age, sex, current weight and level of activity. You will need to recheck this periodically to make sure you can maintain your weight.

In order to add more weight, you must increase this total by 15%. This is easy to do if you add foods that have dense calories to your diet. For example, olive oil is a good fat that has a very high calorie content. Add a tablespoon or two a day.

If your aim is muscle building really fast, these tips will help:

1. You need more calories. At least around 2000 or 2500 calories.

2. Have six meals a day to enable you to eat more and keep up your energy. All meals that you eat should be balanced ones.

3. If your muscles don't seem to be developing as well as you like, or recovery time seems to be too long, you must

make sure that you are getting enough in quality proteins.

4. Try to get a set eating schedule in place. So, try to eat breakfast at the same time every day, ditto for your other meals.

5. Look for healthy fats.

6. Stick to low GI carbs.

7. Make sure that you choose protein sources that are more bioavailable to humans.

8. Find a good multi-vitamin supplement.

9. Choose foods with as close to nature as possible. A good rule of thumb is that if there are more than three or four ingredients, or if there are ingredients you cannot pronounce, you shouldn't be eating it.

If you aim to build a little muscle without the fat, here are some good tips for you:

1. Your total protein intake should be only 0.8 grams for every pound of body weight. You really do not need more.

2. You can increase your calorie intake by around 150 calories a day by including more complex carbs in your diet.

3. If you are still not making headway in terms of weight, add another 150 calories to your daily diet.

Did You Know You Are MOST Likely Burning Fat Too SLOW?

Discover The Most POWERFUL Method to Start Burning Fat Up to 400% Faster!

For this month only, you can get Bruce's best-selling & most popular book absolutely free – *The Most Powerful Method to Burn Fat Up to 400% Faster!*

Get Your FREE Copy Here:
TopFitnessAdvice.com/Download

Discover exactly what you need to do to **put your metabolism into hyperdrive** and have your **fat melt away effortlessly**. And learn the biological "hacks" that have been scientifically proven to **boost the rate that your body burns fat by up to 400%.** With this book, readers were able to reach their fitness goals significantly quicker, so it's highly recommended that you get this book, especially while it's free!

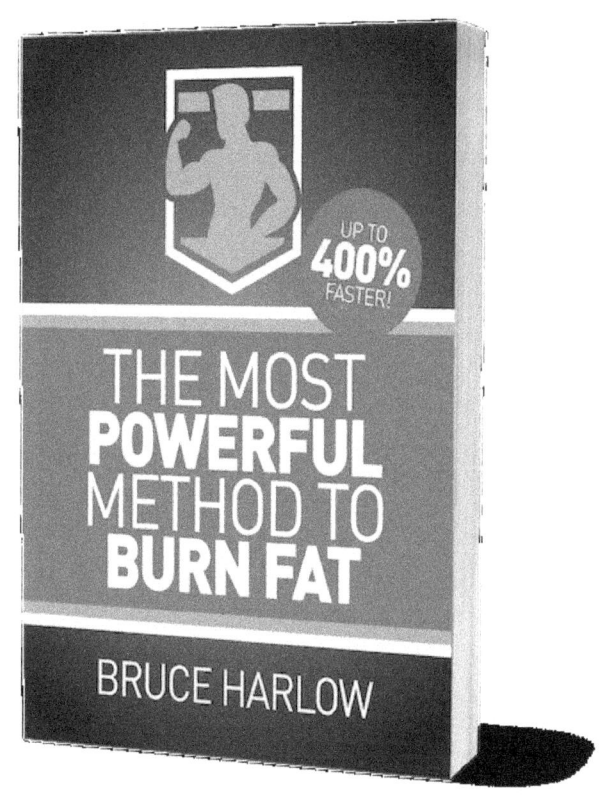

Get Your FREE Copy Here:

TopFitnessAdvice.com/Download

Conclusion

Weight training is both a science and an art. It requires both knowledge and creativity. Your body is your masterpiece. And whatever you do to it is your responsibility.

When engaging in weight training, be sure to be equipped with the knowledge that is contained in this book about effective weight training techniques, some basic nutritional guides, and what not to do to ensure your workout sessions count.

In the end, all this knowledge will only be written on paper and useless unless you apply them. Know the science behind weight training and how to make it work for you. Set your goals right. Plan your training correctly. Execute. Rest well, nourish your body properly, and evaluate the results.

Don't just go to the gym and hit those irons. Don't just sweat for a workout without a direction. Your workouts have to be both fun and effective. Make it count.

Enjoying this book?

Check out our other best sellers!

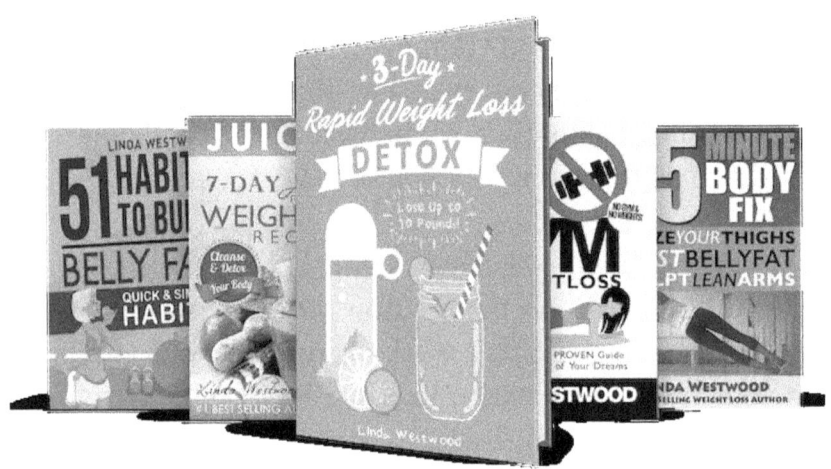

Get your next book on sale here:

TopFitnessAdvice.com/go/books

Final Words

I would like to thank you for purchasing my book and I hope I have been able to help you and educate you on something new.

If you have enjoyed this book and would like to share your positive thoughts, could you please take 30 seconds of your time to go back and give me a review on my Amazon book page.

I greatly appreciate seeing these reviews because it helps me share my hard work.

You can leave me a review on Amazon.com.

Again, thank you and I wish you all the best!

www.ingramcontent.com/pod-product-compliance
Lightning Source LLC
Chambersburg PA
CBHW031156020426
42333CB00013B/685